I0437146

A HANDBOOK OF MULTIVALVULAR AND PROSTHETIC VALVE DISEASE

Alok Ranjan

MD, DNB, MRCP (UK), DM (Card.)
Sr. Consultant - Cardiology
Wockhardt Hospitals
India

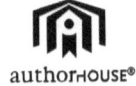

authorHOUSE®

AuthorHouse™
1663 Liberty Drive
Bloomington, IN 47403
www.authorhouse.com
Phone: 1-800-839-8640

© *2012 Alok Ranjan. All rights reserved.*

No part of this book may be reproduced, stored in a retrieval system, or transmitted by any means without the written permission of the author.

Published by AuthorHouse 12/17/2012

ISBN: 978-1-4772-9240-2 (e)
ISBN: 978-1-4772-9241-9 (hc)
ISBN: 978-1-4772-9242-6 (sc)

Library of Congress Control Number: 2012921817

Any people depicted in stock imagery provided by Thinkstock are models, and such images are being used for illustrative purposes only. Certain stock imagery © *Thinkstock.*

This book is printed on acid-free paper.

Because of the dynamic nature of the Internet, any web addresses or links contained in this book may have changed since publication and may no longer be valid. The views expressed in this work are solely those of the author and do not necessarily reflect the views of the publisher, and the publisher hereby disclaims any responsibility for them.

Disclaimer

Medicine is a constantly changing science. New research findings necessitate continual changes in disease concept and its management. The author and publisher of this handbook have used reasonable efforts to provide up-to-date, accurate information that is within generally accepted medical standards at the time of publication. However, as medical science is ever evolving, and human error is always possible, the author and publisher (or any other involved parties) do not guarantee total accuracy or comprehensiveness of the information in this handbook, and they are not responsible for omissions, errors, or the results of using this information. The reader should confirm the accuracy of the information in this handbook from other sources. In particular, all drug doses, indications, and contraindications should be confirmed in package inserts.

The author has made every effort to trace the copyright holders for borrowed material. If he has inadvertently overlooked any, he will be pleased to make necessary arrangement at the first opportunity.

Dedicated to my friends
in Patna Medical College and Hospital

When I go down the memory lane, I am overwhelmed with the memories of time that I have spent with my friends of Patna Medical College. Though I cannot include the names of all of them, a few deserve special mention since they have tolerated me the most; Ashutosh, Amar, Rajat, (Late) Ashish and (Late) Amitabh. I treasure the time spent with them.

"It's the times we're so crazy,
that people think we're high.
It's the times we laugh so hard,
we can't help but cry.
It's all the inside jokes
and "remember whens".
those are all the reasons
that we're best friends!"
- <u>Unknown</u>

Contents

Multivalvular Disease 1

    General concepts 3

    Etiology. 9

    Mixed Single-Valve Disease 11

    Multivalvular lesions. 17

    Tricuspid valve in combined valvular disease. 25

    Pulmonary valve disease in combined valvular disease 29

Prosthetic Valves 33

    Introduction. 35

    Classification of Prosthetic Heart Valves. 37

    Features of commonly used prosthetic valves. 41

    Hemodynamics of prosthetic valves. .53

    Selection of a prosthetic valve 55

    Pre Operative Considerations 56

    Post Operative Considerations 57

    Radiological Appearance of Prosthetic valves. 59

    Follow Up Visits. 60

Prosthetic valve dysfunction 61

    Complications of Prosthetic Valves 65

    Hemorrhagic complications of anticoagulation 67

    Prosthetic thrombosis. 69

    Prosthetic valve endocarditis (PVE). 73

    Hemolysis 77

    Structural Failure of Prosthetic Valves. 79

Prosthetic valve evaluation: Echocardiography 85

Antithrombotic Therapy after prosthetic valve surgery. 97

Pregnancy and Prosthetic Valves. 103

Antibiotics Prophylaxis for Infective Endocarditis 113

Suggested Reading. 117

Abbreviations 123

Multivalvular
Disease

General concepts

Steps in clinical decision making in patients with valvular heart disease.
(Rahimtoola SH)

1. Perform a complete clinical evaluation
   History
   Physical Examination
   Routine blood investigations
   ECG
   Chest X-ray
2. Diagnosis and assess severity of disease
   All valves
   Ventricular Function
   Hemodynamic Effects
   Coronary Artery Disease
   Other Cardiovascular Disease
   Effects on other organs
   Other Organ Diseases
3. List questions that need answering
4. Perform test(s) most likely to provide these answers with the following criteria:
   Reliability
   Accuracy
   Lowest risk to patients
   Reasonable (or lowest) cost

5. Review results of test(s) and make an overall assessment of patient
6. Make recommendations regarding management

Description of cardiac murmurs

Description must include following points
    Timing, configuration or shape
    Character
    Length
    Site of best audibility
    Grade
    Selective conduction
    Relation to physiological act or maneuver
    Accompanying features

Classification of Murmurs

Category	Definition
Systolic Murmur	Starts with or after S1 and ends before or at S2
Ejection systolic	Starts after S1 and ends before S2 of that side (A2 or P2)
Pansystolic	Starts with S1 and ends with S2 of that side (A2 or P2)
Late systolic	Starts after S1 and ends S2 of that side (A2 or P2)
Early systolic	Starts with S1 and does not reach S2

* In the auscultation of systolic murmurs, concentration on the last 1/3rd of systole is of great importance

Diastolic murmurs	Stars with or after S2 and ends at or before S1
Early Diastolic	Starts with S2 (A2 or P2), duration in diastole is variable
Mid diastolic	Starts after S2 and ends before S1
Late diastolic	Starts late after S2 and extends to the S1 of that side (M1 or T1)
Holodiastolic	Occupying whole of diastole from S2 to S1
Continuous murmur	Beginning anywhere in systole, continues into diastole, encompassing S2

Grading of murmurs

Grade I	Faint murmur; Heard on careful examination
Grade II	Easily audible
Grade III	Loud murmur but without thrill
Grade IV	Loud murmur associated with thrill
Grade V	Very loud murmur with thrill
Grade VI	Murmur audible with stethoscope half an inch away from the chest

Character of murmur / sounds

High frequency (High pitch)

Mechanism:	Due to high pressure difference between two chambers
Characteristics:	High numbers of vibrations but of less amplitude Less palpable or have thrills but widely radiated
Description:	Soft / Blowing / Musical / Cooing
Example:	MR (LV – LA pressure difference) AR (AO – LV EDP difference)

Low frequency (Low pitch)

Mechanism:	Low pressure gradient between 2 sites
Characteristics:	Less number of vibrations per second Increased amplitude of vibrations

	Hence, often palpable or have thrills but not well radiated
Description;	Rough / Rumbling / Dull / Thud
Example:	MS (LA to LVEDP difference)
	TS (RA to RVEDP difference)

Mixed frequency (combination)

Mechanism:	High pressure difference between 2 sites
Characteristics:	Combination of frequencies
	Low frequency component is localized to site of best audibility and high frequency is widely radiated
Character:	Harsh / Rough
Example:	AS (Pressure difference between LV and AO)
	PS (Pressure difference between RV and PA)
	VSD (Pressure difference between LV and RV)
	PDA (Pressure difference between AO and PA)

Mechanism of heart sounds

S1: Abrupt termination of movement of elastic coapted cusps of AV valves causes them to stretch and recoil in a rapid vibratory movement.

S2: Rapid force of aortic or pulmonary elastic recoil causes coapted cusps to be tensed and vibrates producing S2

S3: Rapid ventricular filling, which is suddenly halted in situations where the early compliance of LV chamber is decreased.

S4: Forcible atrial contraction against a non compliant ventricle.

Clicks

Ejection click (EC)

Valvular EC: Doming motion of semilunar valve coming to an abrupt halt. Doming is present due to stenosis or deformity of valve.

Vascular EC: Sudden distension of the vessel beyond the valve due to opening of valve

Non – ejection click:

Sounds occurring at AV valves in prolapse of MV or TV due to myxomatous degeneration of valve.

Grade of left parasternal heave

Grade I: Mild lift made out after careful observation or looking at the chest from a tangential view
Grade II: An obvious heave
Grade III: Prominent heave and difficult to suppress
Grade IV: Heave cannot be suppressed

Etiology

Common causes of multivalvular involvement:
  Rheumatic heart disease
  Connective tissue disorders (Mainly regurgitant lesions)
      Marfan's syndrome
      Ehlers Danlos Syndrome
      Others: e.g., SLE (Systemic lupus erythematosus)
  Carcinoid disease
  Myocardial dysfunction disorders (Cardiac remodeling / dilatation)
      Ischemic heart disease
      Dilated cardiomyopathy
      Hypertrophic cardiomyopathy
  Degenerative valve calcification: As seen in aging
  Chronic renal failure
  Infective endocarditis and nonbacterial thrombotic endocarditis (NBTE)
  Radiation therapy
  Drugs and physical agents
      Ergot derivative dopamine agonists pergolide and cabergoline
      Methysergide
      Appetite suppressants fenfluramine and dexfenfluramine
          Pathogenesis is suspected to involve serotonin-mediated

abnormal fibrogenesis by means of the 5-HT2B receptors, which are expressed in the fibroblasts of heart valves

*Multiple valve disease is most likely to be due to RHD, and MS in an adult patient is almost always due to RHD. Isolated acquired AS is rarely due to RHD but rather caused by degenerative changes in bicuspid or tricuspid (elderly patients) aortic valves. Even isolated MR is more commonly due to non rheumatic etiology in western countries.

Multivalvar involvement should be suspected if there is deviation from the expected clinical presentation of the most obvious valvular lesion.

In general, severe calcification is associated with and parallels the degree of valvular stenosis, while severely incompetent valves, with the exception of MR due to a calcified mitral annulus may have little or no calcium.

Involvement of valves in rheumatic heart disease

MV > AV > TV > PV

Exposure to high pressure causes accelerated thickening of valve cusps. MV in closed position is exposed to LV systolic pressure. AV in closed position is exposed to diastolic blood pressure (systolic pressure does not cause pressure to valve cusps collapsed against aortic walls). Hence MV is the most commonly affected in rheumatic process. Same explanation is true for TV and PV also.

The literature does not provide evidence for management guidelines of multiple valve disease. It requires individualization in management due to combined hemodynamic disturbances.

Mixed Single-Valve Disease

In mixed mitral or aortic valve disease, one lesion usually predominates over the other, and the pathophysiology resembles that of the pure dominant lesion.

Diagnosis
(1) 2-D And Doppler echocardiographic Studies: Chamber geometry is important in assessing the dominant lesion (stenotic versus regurgitant), which in turn is important in management. For instance, a small left ventricle is inconsistent with chronic severe regurgitation. Doppler interrogation of the aortic and mitral valves with mixed disease should provide a reliable estimate of the transvalvular mean gradient. However, there may be a significant discrepancy between the Doppler-derived maximum instantaneous gradient and catheter peak gradient with mixed aortic valve disease. Exercise hemodynamics derived by Doppler echocardiography have been helpful in management of mixed valve disease

(2) Cardiac Catheterization. Catheterization is often necessary to fully assess hemodynamics. Although "moderate" mixed disease can be diagnosed on noninvasive tests, but they may not define the indication of surgery. Moderate lesions may not fulfill the criteria of need of surgery. It is well known that coexistent non dominant lesion can worsen the pathophysiology of dominant lesion and

produce symptoms. Such cases may require a complete hemo-dynamic evaluation including exercise hemodynamics to decide about need of intervention. For example, resting hemodynamics in mixed mitral disease might show a transmitral gradient of 8 mm Hg, a valve area of 1.3 cm2, and moderate (2+/3) MR with a resting pulmonary artery wedge pressure of 15 mm. However, with exercise, the wedge pressure may increase to higher levels and explain the patient's symptoms and need of intervention. Many cases of mixed valve disease require hemodynamic exercise testing to delineate proper assessment. Hemodynamic estima-tion of valve area requires determination of total valve flow and transvalvular gradient. The presence of valvular regurgitation in a primarily stenotic valve causes forward cardiac output to underestimate total valve flow, which is the sum of forward plus regurgitant flow. Thus, if standard measures of forward cardiac output (thermodilution, Fick, etc) are used to calculate valve area, the area will be underestimated. One approach to this problem is to use total stroke volume (angiographic end-diastolic volume–end systolic volume) in place of forward stroke volume (Fick or thermodilution cardiac output/heart rate) in the Gorlin formula. The accurate calculation of cardiac volumes may be difficult in the very large and/or spherical left ventricles encountered in valvular regurgitation. In general, the utility of this approach is limited. Doppler pressure half-time may be very useful in this situation.

Management

Unlike the management of a severe pure valve lesion, solid guidelines for mixed disease are difficult to establish. The most logical ap-proach is to correct disease that produces more than mild symptoms or, in the case of AS-dominant aortic valve disease, to operate in the presence of even mild symptoms. In regurgitant dominant lesions, surgery can be delayed until symptoms develop or asymptomatic LV dysfunction (as gauged by markers used in pure regurgitant disease) becomes apparent.

Aortic stenosis with aortic regurgitation

Common Causes:

RHD

Congenital heart disease

Includes supra, valvular and subvalvular stenosis

Bicuspid Aortic valve

Degenerative Aortic disease

HCM: AR is present in 10 % cases of HOCM.

IE

Pathophysiology

Mixed AS and AR where stenosis predominates, the pathophysiology and management resemble that of pure AS. The left ventricle develops concentric hypertrophy rather than dilatation. The timing of AVR is based on symptomatic status. However, if the attendant regurgitation is more than mild, it complicates the pathophysiology by placing the concentrically hypertrophied and noncompliant left ventricle on a steeper portion of its diastolic pressure-volume curve, in turn causing pulmonary congestion. The effect is that neither lesion by itself might be considered severe enough to warrant surgery, but both together produce substantial hemodynamic compromise requiring intervention.

Severe AR and mild AS: The high total stroke volume due to extensive regurgitation may produce a substantial transvalvular gradient. Because the transvalvular gradient varies with the square of the transvalvular flow a high gradient in predominant regurgitation may be predicated primarily on excess transvalvular flow rather than on a severely compromised orifice area.

Features supporting predominant AS:

Presenting symptom

Syncope

Angina

Sustained apex beat

Carotid impulse: Slow upstroke and an early (lower) anacrotic shoulder

Prolonged ejection systolic murmur and wide radiation

Paradoxical split of S2

Soft A2

Predominant AR

Presenting symptoms

Effort intolerance

Dyspnea at rest

Angina

Prolonged EDM

Brisk carotid stroke

Wide pulse pressure

Cardiomegaly with palpable S3

*S3: Presence of S3 in a case of AS always indicates significant coexisting regurgitation

Diagnosis: The aortic valve area can be measured more accurately by the continuity equation from Doppler echocardiography in mixed AS/AR. However, the continuity equation calculation of valve area may not be completely independent of flow. The valve area measurements by Doppler echocardiography are more accurate than those obtained at cardiac catheterization, if cardiac output is measured by either thermodilution or the Fick method on catheterization

Therapy

Mixed AV disease (Rheumatic etiology): AVR

In congenital heart disease where AS is severe and AR is mild: BAV may be considered.

Mitral stenosis with mitral regurgitation

Pathophysiology

In mixed mitral disease, predominant MS produces a left ventricle of normal volume, whereas predominant MR chamber dilatation occurs. A substantial transvalvular gradient may exist in regurgitation-predominant disease because of high transvalvular flow, but (as in mixed aortic valve disease with predominant regurgitation) the gradient does not represent severe orifice stenosis.

Following points indicate a dominant MR:

Easy fatigability

Hyperdynamic apex and LVVO

S1: Soft / Normal

No OS

LV S3

Short MDM with no PSA

Loud PSM at apex with systolic thrill (Grade 4 murmur indicates more than grade 3 MR in 60 % cases)

Following points indicate a dominant MS:

Early development of cough, hemoptysis and pulmonary edema

Early parasternal lift

Long MDM with PSA

Absence of LV enlargement

Loud S1 and prominent OS

Diagnosis: Mitral valve area can be measured accurately by the half-time method in mixed MS/MR.

Therapy:

Anticoagulants should be used in mixed mitral disease if atrial fibrillation is present.

Mixed mitral valve disease with predominant MS: BMV wherever feasible.

In mixed mitral disease with moderate or severe (3+ or 4+) regurgitation, percutaneous mitral balloon valvotomy is contraindicated because regurgitation may worsen.

Mixed mitral valve with predominant MR: MVR

Multivalvular lesions

Mitral stenosis with aortic regurgitation

Pathophysiology

In most cases, severe mitral stenosis coexists with mild aortic regurgitation but aortic regurgitation may be severe. Severe mitral stenosis and aortic regurgitation produce confusing pathophysiology. MS restricts LV filling, blunting the impact of AR on LV volume. Thus, even severe AR may fail to cause a hyperdynamic circulation, so that typical signs of AR are modified during physical examination. The complex combination requires echocardiography and cardiac catheterization for diagnosis. As in clinical features the echocardiographic manifestations may be confusing. LV cavitary dimensions may be only mildly enlarged. Doppler half-time measurements of mitral valve area may be inaccurate in the presence of significant AR.

● Predominant MS: Suggested by
Presence of pulmonary symptoms / emboli
Absence of angina
Absence of peripheral signs of AR
Presence of AF
Presence of loud S1 / OS / PH / Long MDM

Absence of LVVO / Hyperkinetic apex / S3 / S4
- Predominant AR: Suggested by
    Absence of pulmonary symptoms
    Presence of angina
    Peripheral signs of AR
    Presence of EDM / Austin Flint murmur / S3
    Presence of LVVO / Hyperkinetic apex
    Absence of PH / AF / RVH

Severe MS does not mask signs of AR unless patient is in RHF.

Indications for intervention

Symptoms and pulmonary hypertension are usual indications for intervention.

Management
    Options:
        Predominant MS:
            MS suitable for BMV
                BMV and follow up for AR
            MS not suitable for BMV
                MVR +/- AVR,
        Predominant AR
                AVR +/- OMV / MVR.
        Both require attention
                DVR or AVR + OMV.

Mitral stenosis with aortic stenosis

Pathophysiology

The combined valve stenosis is usually rheumatic in origin. Obstruction of flow at the mitral valve diminishes aortic valve flow as well. Thus, the problem of evaluating aortic valve severity in a low flow–low gradient situation often exists.

- Predominant MS: Suggested by
  - Presence of pulmonary symptoms / emboli
  - Absence of angina /syncope
  - Presence of AF
  - Presence of loud S1 / OS / PH / Long MDM
  - Absence of S4 / heaving apex / prominent ESM
- Predominant AS: Suggested by
  - Absence of pulmonary symptoms
  - Presence of angina /syncope
  - Presence of long ESM / S4 / LVH
  - Apex – carotid impulse: Delayed upstroke of impulse
  - Presence of short MDM / prolong A2 – OS gap
  - Absence of PH / AF / RVH

*Whenever the S4 or S3 sounds are palpable, an AV valve stenosis on that side of the heart is unlikely, as neither the presystolic impulse nor the rapid filling of the ventricle are possible with MS or TS.

Diagnosis

Two-dimensional and Doppler echocardiography are performed to assess the severity of aortic stenosis and mitral stenosis, with evaluation of mitral stenosis for mitral balloon valvotomy, and to determine ventricular size and function.

Therapy

> Severe AS with MS where intervention on both valves are required
>> AVR +MVR OR OMV
>
> Severe MS with lesser degree of AS
>> BMV if feasible and follow up for AS
>>
>> MVR if BMV is contraindicated and to decide about AVR on visual inspection or preoperative TEE
>>
>> Severe AS with lesser degree of MS
>>> AVR with OMV if feasible.

Mitral regurgitation with aortic regurgitation

Least common of all combination

Pathophysiology.

> As noted in the previous discussions of isolated MR and AR, these are 2 very different diseases with different pathophysiological effects and different guidelines for the timing of surgery. Thus, in the patient with double valve regurgitation, proper management becomes problematic. The most straightforward approach is the same as for mixed single valve disease, ie, to determine which lesion is dominant and to treat primarily according to that lesion. Although both lesions produce LV dilatation, AR will produce modest systemic systolic hypertension and a mild increase in LV wall thickness.

- Predominant MR: Suggested by
  - Decapitation of SBP
  - LA rock
  - Signs of PH / AF
  - Presence of pulmonary symptoms
- Predominant AR: Suggested by
  - Peripheral signs of AR

- SBP > 140
- DBP < 40
- PP > 50 % SBP

Long EDM with flow murmur

Presence of S4

Diagnosis: Doppler echocardiographic examination shows bivalve regurgitation and an enlarged left ventricle. 2-D echocardiography is usually performed to assess severity of AR and MR, LV size and function, left atrial size, pulmonary artery pressure, and feasibility of mitral valve repair.

Management:

If both lesions are severe, double valve replacement is required.

Severe AR and lesser degree of MR:

Mild to moderate mitral regurgitation may occur secondary to LV dysfunction in chronic, severe aortic regurgitation (as well as stenosis). It may then improve after AVR and coexistent mitral replacement or repair may not then be indicated. If the mitral regurgitation is more than moderate, or if the mitral valve has signs of organic disease, coexistent mitral surgery is necessary.

Severe MR with lesser degree of AR:

MVR and intraoperative TEE to decide about AVR

Mitral regurgitation with aortic stenosis

Pathophysiology

Combined AS and MR often develop secondary to rheumatic heart disease. However, congenital AS and MVP may occur in combination in younger patients, as may degenerative AS and MR in the elderly. If severe, AS will worsen the degree of MR. In addition, MR may cause difficulty in assessing severity of AS because of reduced forward flow. MR will also enhance LV ejection performance, thereby masking the early development of LV systolic dysfunction caused by AS. Development of atrial fibrillation and loss of atrial systole may further reduce forward output because of impaired filling of the hypertrophied left ventricle.

- Predominant MR: Suggested by
  Easy fatigability / pulmonary symptoms
  LA rock / LVVO
  Hyperkinetic apex
  Signs of PH / AF
  Presence of S3 & absence of S4
- Predominant AS: Suggested by
  Angina / syncope
  Delayed carotid upstroke / Heaving apex
  Presence of S4 & absence of S3
  Long and late peaking ESM

Diagnosis

Noninvasive evaluation should be performed with 2-D and Doppler echocardiography to evaluate the severity of both AS and MR. Attention should be paid to LV size, wall thickness and function, left atrial size, right-heart function, and pulmonary artery pressure. Particular attention should be paid to mitral valve morphology in patients with these combined lesions.

Therapy

Patients with severe AS and severe MR (with abnormal mitral valve morphology)
  Combined AVR and MVR or mitral valve repair.
Patients with severe AS and lesser degrees of MR in whom surgery on aortic valve is indicated
  AVR, particularly when there is normal mitral valve morphology.

Intraoperative transesophageal echocardiography and, if necessary, visual inspection of the mitral valve should be performed at the time of AVR to determine whether additional mitral valve surgery is warranted in these patients.

Patients with mild to moderate AS and severe MR in whom surgery on the mitral valve is indicated

MVR

Preoperative assessment of the severity of AS may be difficult because of reduced forward stroke volume.

If the mean aortic valve gradient is .more than 30 mm Hg, AVR should be performed.

In patients with less severe aortic valve gradients, inspection of the aortic valve and its degree of opening on 2-D or transesophageal echocardiography as well as visual inspection by the surgeon may be important in determining the need for concomitant AVR.

Tricuspid valve in combined valvular disease

Tricuspid Stenosis in combined valvular disease

Rheumatic TS almost always coexist with mitral stenosis. It is rarely present with predominant MR

Features raising suspicion of TS in a patient with known mitral and / or aortic valve disease:
    Lack of acute paroxysmal symptoms: Such as
        PND
        Severe pulmonary edema
        Sudden massive hemoptysis
    Relative paucity of pulmonary symptoms (proposed by Gibson and Wood)
    Typical symptoms of TS (due to diminished cardiac output)
        Easy fatigability
        Effort intolerance
    Signs:
        JVP
          Giant 'A' waves with slow 'y' descent
        Absence of parasternal lift
        Split S1

MDM at tricuspid area: Inspiratory augmentation of murmur (described by Carvallo)
* If both TS and TR murmurs are present, inspiratory augmentation of diastolic murmur and reduction of systolic murmur indicate dominant TS.

ECG:

Tall, peaked 'P' wave without evidence of RVH (PH)

Prolonged PR interval

Delay in intratrial conduction

Diminutive RSr' complex in V1-V2 associated with P wave of larger amplitude than QRS amplitude

*Highly suggestive of TS

CXR:

RAE without prominent pulmonary arteries

Tricuspid regurgitation in combined valvular disease

Isolated rheumatic TR is never present

Features raising suspicion of **organic** TR in a patient with known mitral and / or aortic valve disease

Lack of paroxysmal pulmonary symptoms

PSM at tricuspid area with inspiratory augmentation (Carvallo's sign)

Absence of Carvallo's sign does NOT exclude TR

If both TS and TR murmurs are present, inspiratory augmentation of systolic murmur indicate a dominant TR.

Lack of signs of pulmonary hypertension

Management of Tricuspid Valve Disease in a case of multivalvular involvement

Class I

Tricuspid valve repair is beneficial for severe tricuspid regurgitation (TR) in patients with MV disease requiring MV surgery. *(Level of Evidence: B)*

Class IIa

1. Tricuspid valve replacement or annuloplasty is reasonable for severe primary TR when symptomatic. *(Level of Evidence: C)*
2. Tricuspid valve replacement is reasonable for severe TR secondary to diseased/abnormal tricuspid valve leaflets not amenable to annuloplasty or repair. *(Level of Evidence: C)*

Class IIb

Tricuspid annuloplasty may be considered for less than severe TR in patients undergoing MV surgery when there is pulmonary hypertension or tricuspid annular dilatation. *(Level of Evidence: C)*

Class III

1. Tricuspid valve replacement or annuloplasty is not indicated in asymptomatic patients with TR whose pulmonary artery systolic pressure is less than 60 mm Hg in the presence of a normal MV. *(Level of Evidence: C)*
2. Tricuspid valve replacement or annuloplasty is not indicated in patients with mild primary TR. *(Level of Evidence: C)*

Pulmonary valve disease in combined valvular disease

Rheumatic involvement of PV is extremely uncommon. PV is most uncommon valve to be affected by RHD. Its affection usually indicates a quadrivalvular RHD. Other cause of quadrivalvular involvement is myxomatous degeneration of valves.

Carcinoid disease is one condition where there is predilection for pulmonary valve involvement

Tuberculosis and gonococcal infections are unusual forms of infective endocarditis with a predilection for pulmonary valve involvement.

Characteristics

> The first indication of combined pulmonary valvular disease is on echocardiographic examination

> In cases of severe PH, Graham Steell's murmur can be heard. It can be easily differentiated from AR murmur if peripheral signs of AR are absent. Otherwise, symptoms and signs of pulmonary lesion in combined valve disease is difficult to separate from other valve lesions.

> Ejection pulmonary click is not present in Rheumatic PS.

Classification of the Severity of Valve Disease in Adults

A. Left-sided valve disease			
	Aortic Stenosis		
Indicator	**Mild**	**Moderate**	**Severe**
Jet velocity (m/s)	Less than 3.0	3.0-4.0	Greater than 4.0
Mean gradient (mm Hg)*	Less than 25	25-40	Greater than 40
Valve area (cm²)	Greater than 1.5	1.0-1.5	Less than 1.0
Valve area index (cm²/m²)			Less than 0.6
	Mitral Stenosis		
	Mild	**Moderate**	**Severe**
Mean gradient (mm Hg)*	Less than 5	5-10	Greater than 10
Pulmonary artery systolic pressure (mm Hg)	Less than 30	30-50	Greater than 50
Valve area (cm²)	Greater than 1.5	1.0-1.5	Less than 1.0
	Aortic Regurgitation		
	Mild	**Moderate**	**Severe**
Qualitative			
Angiographic grade	1+	2+	3-4+
Color Doppler jet	Central jet, width less than 25% of LVOT	Greater than mild but no signs of severe AR	Central jet, width greater than 65% LVOT
Doppler vena contracta width (cm)	Less than 0.3	0.3-0.6	Greater than 0.6
Quantitative (cath or echo)			
Regurgitant volume (ml/beat)	Less than 30	30-59	Greater than or equal to 60
Regurgitant fraction (%)	Less than 30	30-49	Greater than or equal to 50
Regurgitant orifice area (cm²)	Less than 0.10	0.10-0.29	Greater than or equal to 0.30
Additional Essential Criteria			
Left ventricular size			Increased

A. Left-sided valve disease			
	Aortic Stenosis		
Indicator	**Mild**	**Moderate**	**Severe**
	Mitral Regurgitation		
	Mild	**Moderate**	**Severe**
Qualitative			
Angiographic grade	1+	2+	3-4+
Color Doppler jet width	Small, central jet (less than 4 cm² or less than 20% LA area)	Signs of MR greater than mild present but no criteria for severe MR	Vena contracta width greater than 0.7 cm with large central MR jet (area greater than 40% of LA area) or with a wall-impinging jet of any size, swirling in LA
Doppler vena contracta width (cm)	Less than 0.3	0.3-0.69	Greater than or equal to 0.70
Quantitative (cath or echo)			
Regurgitant volume (ml/beat)	Less than 30	30-59	Greater than or equal to 60
Regurgitant fraction (%)	Less than 30	30-49	Greater than or equal to 50
Regurgitant orifice area (cm²)	Less than 0.20	0.20-0.39	Greater than or equal to 0.40
Additional Essential Criteria			
Left atrial size			Enlarged
Left ventricular size			Enlarged
B. Right-Sided Valve Disease	**Characteristic**		
Severe tricuspid stenosis:	Valve area less than 1.0 cm²		
Severe tricuspid regurgitation:	Vena contracta width greater than 0.7 cm and systolic flow reversal in hepatic veins		
Severe pulmonic stenosis:	Jet velocity greater than 4 m/s or maximum gradient greater than 60 mm Hg		
Severe pulmonic regurgitation:	Color jet fills outflow tract; dense continuous wave Doppler signal with a steep deceleration slope		

*Valve gradients are flow dependent and when used as estimates of severity of valve stenosis should be assessed with knowledge of cardiac output or forward flow across the valve. Modified from Zoghbi WA, Enriquez-Sarano M, Foster E, et al. Recommendations for evaluation of the severity of native valvular regurgitation with two-dimensional and Doppler echocardiography. J Am Soc Echocardiogr 2003;16:777–802 (27).

AR = aortic regurgitation; cath = catheterization; echo = echocardiography; LA = left atrial/atrium; LVOT = left ventricular outflow tract; MR = mitral regurgitation.

Prosthetic Valves

History

Cardiopulmonary bypass machine: Gibbon; 1953

Mitral valve replacement: Starr and Edwards; 1960

Aortic valve replacement: Harken et al; 1960

Carpentier introduced the treatment of tissue valve with glutaraldehyde

Tilting disc introduced in 1969

Bileaflet valve introduced in 1979

First bioprosthetic valve: Hancock porcine valve was available in 1970.

Introduction

Dwight Harken's Ten Commandments for ideal prosthetic valves

Chemically inert; does not damage blood elements

Offer no resistance to physiological flow

Must close promptly (< 0.05 sec)

Must remain close during appropriate phase of cardiac cycle

Have lasting physical geometric features

Inserted in a physiological site

Must not propagate emboli

Capable of permanent fixation

Must not annoy the patient

Technically practical to insert

* All prosthetic valves are inherently obstructive and have a significantly smaller valve area than the normal native valves.

Classification of Prosthetic Heart Valves

- Mechanical prostheses:
  - Rigid, manufactured occluders
- Biological or tissue valves :
  - With flexible leaflet occluders of animal or human origin
- Percutaneous implantable prosthetic valves
    Emerging as an alternative to standard valve replacement.

Mechanical Valves

1. *Ball in cage*
    Starr-Edwards valve: Discontinued in 2007
    Braunwald-Cutter: Discontinued

2. Disc in cage: Lower profile and high flow resistance
    Discontinued
3. *Tilting disc valves*: Uses a circular disc as an occluder
    Bjork – Shiley (Discontinued), Medtronic Hall, Shri Chitra

4. *Bileaflet Disc Valves*: The 2 semicircular leaflets of a bileaflet
    valve are connected to the orifice housing by a butterfly hinge
    mechanism.
    St. Judes, Sorin, Omniscience

Biological (Tissue) Valves:

The term bioprosthesis is used for a nonviable tissue of biological origin

Autograft valve: refers to a translocation within the same individual, e.g., of the pulmonary valve into the aortic valve position.

Autologous (or autogenous) tissue valve: involves fabricating a valve from the patient's own nonvalvular tissue, e.g., pericardium.

Homograft (or allograft) valve: refers to transplantation from a donor of the same species; e.g., a donor's aortic or pulmonary valve into a recipient's aortic or pulmonary position.

Heterograft (or xenograft) valve: is a transplant from another species, either an intact valve, e.g., a porcine aortic valve, or a valve fashioned from heterologous tissue, e.g., bovine pericardium.

Advantages:
Reduces the complications associated with thromboembolism
No need for anticoagulation
In the aortic position to optimize hemodynamics

Examples of biological valves:
a. Autograft Valves
   Ross procedure: Pulmonary autograft in aortic position and valve prosthesis at pulmonary position.
b. Autologous Valves: Made from patient's own pericardium.
   Frame-mounted autologous pericardial valve.
c. Homograft (or Allograft) Valves: Cadaver valves
   Excellent hemodynamics
   Low thrombogenicity
   No need for anticoagulation.

Drawbacks:

Technically demanding operation

Structural deterioration is fast: The newer antibiotic treated cryopreserved frozen irradiated
valves have similar rate of structural deterioration as compared to porcine valves

Low availability.

d.Heterograft or Xenograft:

Porcine Heterograft (or Xenograft) Valves.

Glutaraldehyde sterilized valve tissue

Made bioacceptable by destroying antigenicity

Stabilizes the collagen crosslinks for durability

Examples:

Hancock and

Carpentier-Edwards porcine valves

Bovine Pericardial Valves.

Pericardial valves are tailored and sewn into
a valvular configuration on a stented frame,
with bovine pericardium as a fabric.

Better hemodynamics.

Greater durability

Examples:

Ionescu-Shiley,

Carpentier-Edwards Pericardial Bioprosthesis

FDA-Approved Prosthetic Heart Valves

Type	Manufacturer	Model
Mechanical		
Ball	Baxter Edwards	Starr-Edwards
Disc	Medtronic	Medtronic Hall
	Medical Inc.	Omniscience
	Alliance	Monostrut
Bileaflet	St. Jude	St. Jude
	Baxter Edwards	Duromedics
	CarboMedics	CarboMedics
Biological		
Porcine	Medtronic	Hancock Standard
		Hancock MO•
	Baxter Edwards	CE■ Standard
		CE■ SupraAnnular
	St. Jude	Toronto Stentless
	Medtronic	Free Style Stentless
Pericardial	Baxter Edwards	CE■
Homograft	noncommercial	
	Cryolife	
Autologous	noncommercial	Pulmonary autograft

•MO modified orifice, ■CE Carpentier-Edwards

40

Features of commonly used prosthetic valves

Starr – Edwards valve:

    Type: Caged ball

        Ball: Forms central occluder: Responsible for 'bulky' design

            Made of silicone rubber

        Cage: Limits movement of ball

            Made of 3 -4 struts (may or may not be joined at apex) that project from the inner ring on the outflow surface

      Struts: Stellite alloy

      Sewing ring: Teflon / polypropylene cloth

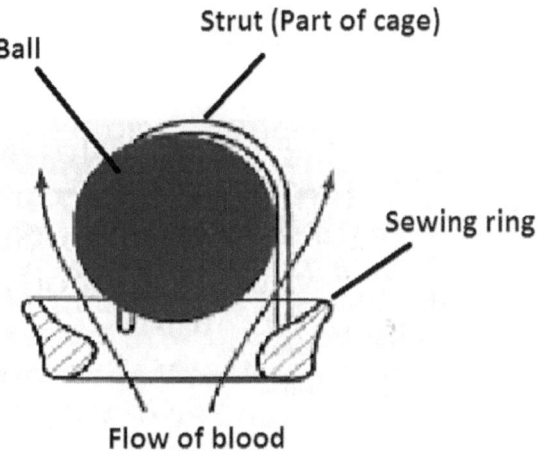

41

Advantages:

Longest track record of reliability and durability

Disadvantages:

Lifelong anticoagulation is essential

Hemolysis

Poor hemodynamics in small sizes

Normal auscultatory findings in patients with caged – ball valves:

Caged – ball in Mitral position

Findings

S1: Always abnormal, as it is produced by prosthetic valve

Produced by closing of prosthetic valve hence called as 'mitral closing' sound (MC)

Sharp metallic sound

S2: Normal as it is produced by native semilunar valves. Any abnormality in these valves will alter S2. For example loud P2 in presence of PH

Mitral opening sound (MO):

Produced by opening of metallic valve, this co-incides with maximum excursion of 'ball prosthesis'

Similar in duration of A2-OS gap of moderate MS (0.07 – 0.13 sec)

Any prolongation or reduction of A2 – MO interval suggests prosthetic dysfunction.

In caged-ball prosthesis MO is louder than MC

Murmur:

Systolic murmur

Common

Early to mid systolic murmur

Heard at apex or at lower sternal border

Not due to prosthetic regurgitation

Probably related to turbulence produced by projection of rigid prosthetic cage into LVOT

Diastolic murmur:

Not present

Its presence in cage-ball valve always represents prosthetic dysfunction

Presystolic sounds produced by atrial systole causing motion of ball into cage are not audible.

Caged – ball in Aortic position

Findings

S1:   Normal, as it is produced by AV valves

S2:   Abnormal

A2 is produced by aortic closing (AC) sound of prosthetic valve

Less loud than the aortic opening (AO) sound

Aortic opening sound (AO):

Produced by opening of metallic valve, this coincides with maximum excursion of 'ball prosthesis'

S1 – AO gap: 0.07 sec

In caged-*ball prosthesis AO is louder than AC*

AO to AC amplitude ratio (on phonocardiogram) is > 0.5. Reduction of this ratio is suggestive of ball valve dysfunction

However, preservation of this ratio does not exclude ball valve dysfunction

Murmur:

Systolic murmur

Common

Ejection systolic murmur

Heard at base and may radiate to carotids

Related to turbulence caused by 'normal' prosthetic gradients

Diastolic murmur:

Not present

Its presence in cage-ball valve always represents prosthetic dysfunction

Disc Valve:

Introduced in mid 1960s

Referred as low profile valve

Caged disc: Similar in concept to caged ball but here a disc is present in place of ball; it allows for a **smaller cage**

Higher thrombogenicity than cage-ball valve

Tilting disc (single or bileaflet discs)

Advantages:

Smaller size

Low profile

Good hemodynamics even in smaller sizes

Good durability

Disadvantages:

Lifelong anticoagulation

Sudden and catastrophic valve thrombosis

Starr Edward caged disc valve:

Type: Caged disc

Occluder:

Disc; Single (oscillates in closed and open position)

Sits on a ring in closed position and oscillates away from the ring in open position (pivots on central axis)

Struts:

Open or closed metal struts

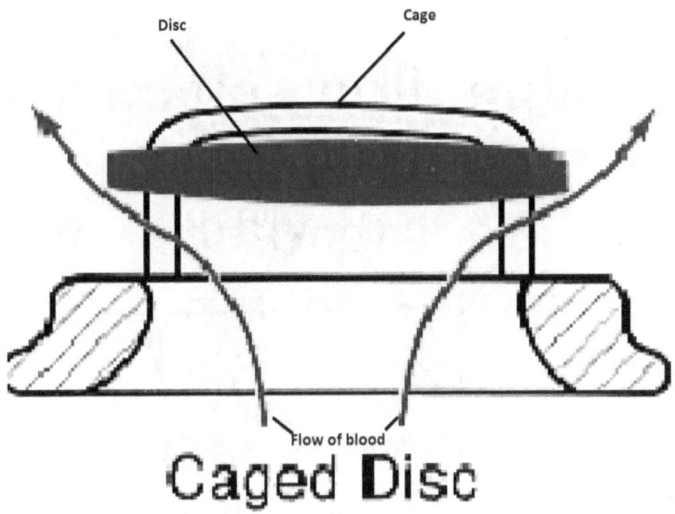

Caged Disc

Tilting disc:

    Occluder:

        Disc; Single (oscillates in closed and open position)

            The opening angle of the disk relative to valve annulus ranges from 60° to 80°, resulting in 2 distinct orifices of different sizes

            Opens to provide a major and minor orifice for blood flow.

                Wider the 'opening angle' more laminar is the flow and lower is the flow differences

    Struts:

        Open or closed metal struts

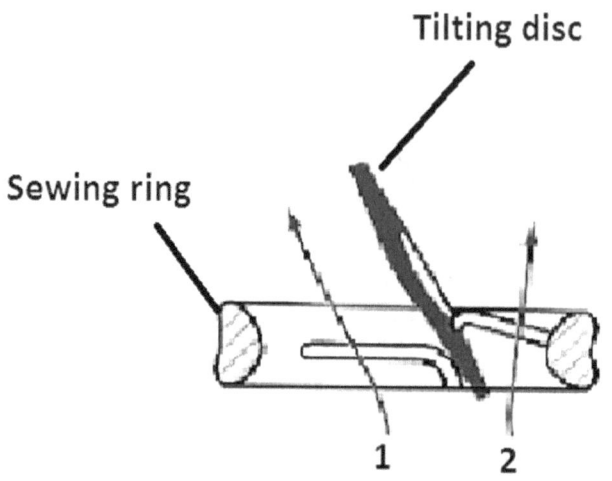

Tilting disc

Sewing ring

1   2

Flow of blood
1.: Major orifice
2.: Minor orifice

Omniscience:
> Type: Tilting disc
>> Pyrolytic carbon coated disc within titanium housing with a polyester knit sewing Ring

*Pyrolytic carbon prevents 'fatigue failure' of mechanical valves. Fatigue failure is due to polycrystalline characteristics of metals and prolific carbon is not crystalline in nature

Medtronic Hall valve:
> Type: Tilting disc
>> Pyrolytic carbon coated disc within titanium housing with Teflon sewing ring
>> Disc has central perforation to provide improved hemodynamics

Bileaflet disc valve
> *St. Jude Bileaflet valve:*

Type: Bileaflet disc
Occluder: 2 semicircular discs
Discs pivot between open and closed position]
The opening angle of the leaflets relative to the an-
nulus plane ranges from 75° to 90°
Open valve consists of 3 orifices: a small, slit-like cen-
tral orifice between the 2 open leaflets and 2 larger
semicircular orifices laterally.
Discs are coated with pyrolytic carbon
No need of supporting struts

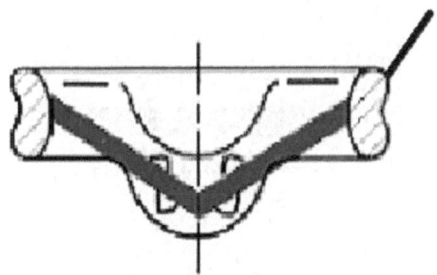

Bileaflet tilting disc in closed position

Bileaflets in open position

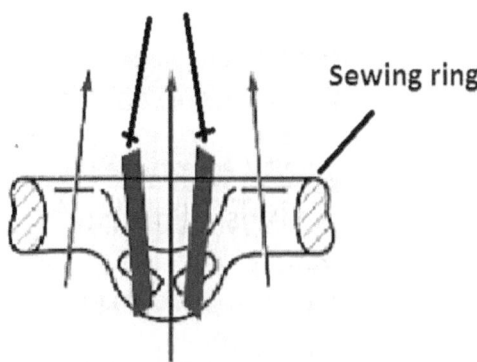

**Flow of blood with 2 lateral
and 1 central jets**

Carbomedics prosthesis:
> Variation of St. Jude bileaflet valve
>
> Pyrolytic carbon coated discs with titanium housing

Normal auscultatory findings in disc valves:

In Mitral position
> Findings
>> S1: Always abnormal, as it is produced by prosthetic valve
>>
>> Produced by closing of prosthetic valve hence called as 'mitral closing' sound (MC)
>>
>> Sharp metallic sound
>>
>> S2: Normal as it is produced by native semilunar valves. Any abnormality in these valves will alter S2. For example loud P2 in presence of PH
>>
>> Mitral opening sound (MO):
>>> Usually not audible, almost absent in bileaflet valves
>>>
>>> The relatively lightweight discs do not strike any resonant structure and hence MO is not prominent in disc valves.

In disc prosthesis only MC is present.

>> Murmur:
>>> Systolic murmur
>>>> Present in tilting disc, unusual in bileaflet valves
>>>>
>>>> Early to mid systolic murmur: $\leq$ 2 grade murmur
>>>>
>>>> Heard at apex or at lower sternal border
>>>>
>>>> Probably related to turbulence produced

by projection of rigid prosthetic cage into LVOT

Diastolic murmur:

Faint (≤ 2 grade) diastolic murmur may be present, less common in bileaflet valve

Due to LA to LV pressure gradient caused by an effective MVA less than half of native mitral valve area produced by these disc valves.

However a prominent MDM should always be suspected to be due to prosthetic dysfunction.

In Aortic position

Findings

S1: Normal, as it is produced by AV valves

S2: Abnormal

A2 is produced by aortic closing (AC) sound of prosthetic valve

Aortic opening sound (AO):

Uncommon, almost never heard in bileaflet valves

S1 – AO gap: 0.04 sec in Tilting disc valve

Murmur:

Systolic murmur

Common in Tilting disc, uncommon in Bileaflet valves

Ejection systolic murmur

Heard at base

Related to turbulence caused by 'normal' prosthetic gradients

Diastolic murmur:

Disc valve
> Its presence almost always represents prosthetic dysfunction

Bioprosthetic valves:
> 3 cusps commonly supported on a frame consisting of a sewing ring and cloth covered struts

Cloth covered struts

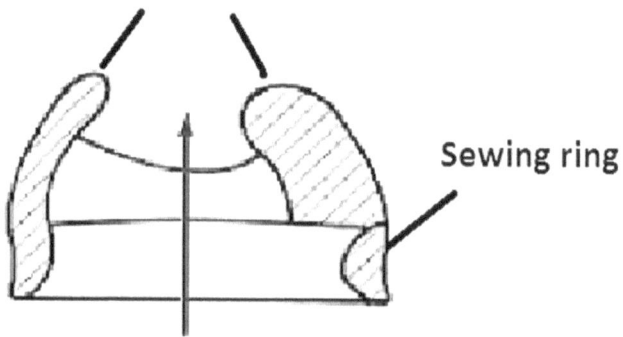

Sewing ring

Flow of blood

Hancock valve:
> Type: Porcine
>> Fixed and preserved in glutaraldehyde
>> Mounted on a Dacron cloth-covered flexible polypropylene strut

Carpentier-Edwards valve
> Type: Porcine
>> Pressure fixed and then preserved in glutaraldehyde
>> Mounted on a Teflon covered Eljiloy strut

Normal auscultatory findings in tissue valves:

Findings		Mitral position	Aortic position
S1		Normal	Normal
	Closing sound	Similar to normal S1	-
	Opening sound	**Opening snap** present (50 %)	
		A2-MO gap: 0.10 sec	
S2		Normal	Normal
	Closing sound		Like normal A2
	Opening sound		Rare
Diastolic murmur		Present in 1/3rd to 2/3rd cases	-
Systolic sound			
	Ejection murmur	Present (50 %)	Present ~ 100 %

Hemodynamics of prosthetic valves

All prosthetic valves are 'stenotic' since the effective in-vivo valve area is less than the normal mitral or aortic valve area. The effective area may diminish further secondary to tissue in growth and endothelialization.

The prosthetic valve regurgitation is minimal. More than mild prosthetic regurgitation or any paraprosthetic regurgitation is considered abnormal.

Type of valve	Mean gradient at rest (mm Hg)	
	Mitral position	Aortic position
Starr-Edwards	3 – 8	10 – 20
Tilting disc	3 – 7	5 – 15
Bileaflet disc	5	5
Bioprosthesis	2 – 8	6 – 23

The gradients tend to increase further with exercise.
The gradients are higher with smaller valves.

Bi-leaflet Valves:

> These valves have a localized, high velocity central jet with rapid pressure recovery distal to the valve.

> > CW Doppler records the highest velocity and thus, the central jet is recorded.

An erroneous diagnosis of severe stenosis may be made.

The central jet reduces with stenosis due to less movement of the leaflets, likely making gradient measurements more accurate.

Helpful if a baseline study was done just after valve replacement (pre discharge)

Selection of a prosthetic valve

Recommendations for Mechanical Prosthesis

Class I

1. Patients with expected long life spans.
2. Patients with a mechanical prosthetic valve already in place in a different position than the valve to be replaced.

Class II

1. Patients in renal failure, on hemodialysis, or with hypercalcemia (Class II)

2. Patients requiring warfarin therapy because of risk factors* for thromboembolism. (Class IIa)

3. Patients ≤ 65 years for AVR and ≤ 70 years for MVR. (Class IIa)

4. Valve rereplacement for thrombosed biological valve. (Class IIb)

*Risk factors: atrial fibrillation, severe LV dysfunction, previous thrombo-embolism, and hypercoagulable condition.

Recommendations for Bioprosthesis

Class I

1. Patients who cannot or will not take warfarin therapy.
2. Patients ≥ 65 years* needing AVR who do not have risk factors for thromboembolism.

Class II

1. Patients considered to have possible compliance problems with warfarin therapy. (Class IIa)
2. Patients >70 years* needing MVR who do not have risk factors for thromboembolism.† (Class IIa)
3. Valve rereplacement for thrombosed mechanical valve. (Class IIb)
4. Patients <65 years.* (Class IIb)

> *The age at which patients should be considered for bioprosthetic valves is based on the major reduction in rate of structural valve deterioration after age 65 and increased   risk of bleeding in this age group.
> †Risk factors: atrial fibrillation, severe LV dysfunction, previous thromboembolism, and hypercoagulable condition

Homograft valve

Female of child bearing age (first choice at aortic position)
Endocarditis
Small aortic root
Any young patient who requires a tissue valve in aortic position
In aortic position if root enlargement is part of aortoventriculoplasty (Konno procedure)

Prosthetic valves: Pre Operative Considerations

Nutritional support
Aggressive diuresis
Measures to prevent respiratory failure
Presence of Atrial Fibrillation
Dental checks: IE prophylaxis
Cardiac catheterization
    To rule associated CAD
        > 40 yrs old patients should be subjected to routine preoperative coronary angiography

If non invasive methods are not accurate in diagnosing the
severity of lesions

Selection of valve type

Counseling

Asymptomatic patients may question the need for such dramatic surgery

Valve choice

Lifestyle changes relating to warfarin therapy

Education regarding endocarditis

Prosthetic valves: Post-operative Considerations

Routine complications post cardiac surgery

Fluid and hemodynamic monitoring and management

Education regarding anticoagulation therapy

Arrhythmias / complete heart block and need for permanent
pacemaker

Symptoms / Dyspnea may take time to improve

Prophylactic antibiotic therapy prior to dental work and other invasive
procedures

Prosthetic valves: Operative mortality

Single valve replacement (Mitral or Aortic)

2 – 10 %

Multiple valve operations

5 – 10 %

10 yr. survival is about 60 % after valve replacement

Valve replacements for stenotic lesions do better than regurgitant
lesions

Radiological Appearance of Prosthetic valves

The following are descriptions of the radiographic appearance of the more commonly seen valves.

Starr-Edwards caged ball valve

- Radiopaque base ring
- Radiopaque cage
- Three struts for the aortic valve; 4 struts for the mitral or tricuspid valve
- Silastic ball impregnated with barium that is mildly radiopaque (but not in all models)

Bjork-Shiley tilting disc valve

- Base ring and struts are radiopaque.
- Two U-shaped struts project into base ring.
- Edge of occluder disc is also radiopaque.

Medtronic-Hall tilting disc valve

- Radiopaque base ring
- Radiopaque struts that project into base ring: 3 small ones and 1 large hook-shaped one
- Occluder disc that is mildly opaque but often cannot be seen

St Jude medical bileaflet valve

- Mildly radiopaque leaflets are best seen when viewed on end.
- Base ring is not visualized on most models.

- The valve may not be visualized on radiograph.

Carpentier-Edwards porcine valve: The tall serpiginous wire support is the only visualized portion.

Hancock porcine valve

- The radiopaque base ring is the only visible part in some models.
- Other models have radiopaque stent markers with or without a visible base ring.

Ionescu-Shiley bovine pericardial valve: Base ring and wide fenestrated stents are one piece.

Prosthetic valves: Follow-Up Visits: Recommendations

Class I

1. For patients with prosthetic heart valves, a history, physical examination, and appropriate tests should be performed at the first postoperative outpatient evaluation, 2 to 4 weeks after hospital discharge. This should include a transthoracic Doppler echocardiogram if a baseline echocardiogram was not obtained before hospital discharge. *(Level of Evidence: C)*
2. For patients with prosthetic heart valves, routine follow-up visits should be conducted annually, with earlier re-evaluations (with echocardiography) if there is a change in clinical status. *(Level of Evidence: C)*

Class IIb

Patients with bioprosthetic valves may be considered for annual echocardiograms after the first 5 years in the absence of a change in clinical status. *(Level of Evidence: C)*

Class III

Routine annual echocardiograms are not indicated in the absence of a change in clinical status in patients with mechanical heart valves or during the first 5 years after valve replacement with a bioprosthetic valve. *(Level of Evidence: C)*

Prosthetic valve dysfunction

Changes in symptoms or physical findings are usually the first signs of prosthetic valve dysfunction. Deterioration of clinical status should always be taken as prosthetic valve dysfunction unless proved otherwise.

Auscultatory findings suggestive of prosthetic valve dysfunction

Findings common to any position of prosthetic valve:

> Absence or definite reduction of a prosthetic opening (OC) or closing click (CC) as previously heard either by doctor or patient
> Change in intensity of OC to CC clicks
> Beat to beat variability in the intensity of OC or CC clicks or random alterations in the timing relationship of prosthetic sounds

Findings with prosthetic valve at mitral position.
> Presence of PSM (pansystolic murmur) at apex
> A prominent MDM at apex or changing or 'new' MDM
> ≤ 2 grade murmur may be a normal finding especially in Bileaflet or bioprosthetic valve
> Either prolonged S2-OS (opening sound) or shortened S2-OS interval
> Prolonged if
> Interference with ball excursion
> Shortened if
> Prosthetic obstruction (< 0.1 msec)
> Severe paravalvular regurgitation

Findings with prosthesis in aortic position
> Presence of long, 'kite' shaped ESM: > grade 2 murmur
> Presence of EDM (early diastolic murmur)
> A faint diastolic murmur may be present in tilting disc valve

*Significant prosthetic dysfunction may be present even without audible changes in valve opening or closing sounds or without pathognomonic murmurs

Complications of Prosthetic Valves

Hemorrhagic complications of anticoagulation

Systemic embolism

Prosthetic valve endocarditis

Hemolysis

Mechanical obstruction

    Obstruction: Valve thrombosis; Valve prosthesis–patient mismatch

    Insufficiency: Disruption of valve leaflets; valve sticking in open position

Paravalvular leaks

Other: Ball variance; ball wear, strut failure, dehiscence

Unusual complications after cardiac valve surgery:

    Pseudoaneurysms of Composite Aortic Grafts

        Seen at the proximal or distal graft anastomosis or at coronary arteries anastomosis sites in Bentall's procedure

    Left Ventricular Pseudoaneurysm after MVR

    Abscess and Pseudoaneurysm of the Mitral-aortic intervalvular Fibrosa

    Intracardiac Fistulas after Valve Replacement

Hemorrhagic complications of anticoagulation

Anticoagulant related bleeding (percent per year)

Fatal: 0.5 %

Major: 1 -2 %

Minor: 4 – 8 %

Age > 70 yrs is at higher risk (9 % per year)

All patients with prosthetic valves (including bioprosthetic valves) should receive anticoagulation for first 3 months after valve surgery. After 3 months, all patients with mechanical valves and patients with bioprosthesis with high risk for valve thrombosis should receive lifelong anticoagulation.

Bridging Therapy in Patients With Mechanical Valves Who Require Interruption of Warfarin Therapy for Noncardiac Surgery, Invasive Procedures, or Dental Care

Class I

1. In patients at low risk of thrombosis, defined as those with a bileaflet mechanical AVR with no risk factors,* it is recommended that warfarin be stopped 48 to 72 hour before the procedure (so the INR falls to less than 1.5) and restarted within 24 h after the procedure. Heparin is usually unnecessary. *(Level of Evidence: B)*

2. In patients at high risk of thrombosis, defined as those with any mechanical MV replacement or a mechanical AVR with any risk factor, therapeutic doses of intravenous UFH should be started when the INR falls below 2.0 (typically 48 h before surgery), stopped 4 to 6 h before the procedure, restarted as early after surgery as bleeding stability allows, and continued until the INR is again therapeutic with warfarin therapy. *(Level of Evidence: **B**)*

Class IIa

It is reasonable to give fresh frozen plasma to patients with mechanical valves who require interruption of warfarin therapy for emergency noncardiac surgery, invasive procedures, or dental care. Fresh frozen plasma is preferable to high-dose vitamin K1. *(Level of Evidence: **B**)*

Class IIb

In patients at high risk of thrombosis (see above), therapeutic doses of subcutaneous UFH (15,000 units every 12 h) or LMWH (100 units per kg every 12 hours) may be considered during the period of a subtherapeutic INR. *(Level of Evidence: **B**)*

Class III

In patients with mechanical valves who require interruption of warfarin therapy for noncardiac surgery, invasive procedures, or dental care, high-dose vitamin K1 should not be given routinely, because this may create a hypercoagulable condition. *(Level of Evidence: **B**)*

*Risk factors: atrial fibrillation, previous thromboembolism, LV dysfunction, hypercoagulable conditions, older generation thrombogenic valves, mechanical tricuspid valves, or more than 1 mechanical valve.

Patients with aortic prosthesis have lower risk of valve thrombosis, however the risk increases significantly 24 hours post discontinuation of anticoagulants.

* If a patient develops recurrent emboli with a mechanical valve despite adequate anticoagulation, replacement with bioprosthesis is recommended.

Prosthetic Valve thrombosis:

Thromboembolism
  Mitral position: 2 – 5 % per patient year
  Aortic position: 1 – 2 % per patient year
  Mechanical valve: 2 – 4 % per patient year
  Bioprosthetic valve: 1 – 2 % per patient year

Valve thrombosis: Mortality about 50 %
  Site of prosthesis:
        Prosthesis at tricuspid position has the highest and at aortic position has the least chance of thrombosis
        (TV > MV > AV)
  Type of prosthesis:
        Mechanical > Bioprosthesis
          In mechanical valves:
                Bjork – Shiley and Starr Edwards > Others
  Reasons:
        Prosthesis factors:
                Prosthesis may cause turbulence, shearing stress, stagnation, eddy currents that may damage cellular elements and release factors that evoke the normal clotting reaction.
        Valve materials may encourage thrombosis (cloth struts have higher chance of thrombosis than unclothe ones)
        Patient factors:
                Drug non compliance: Most frequent cause in Indian subsets

High risk conditions for thrombosis
   Risk factors: Atrial fibrillation, LV dysfunction, previous
   thromboembolism, and hypercoagulable condition

Thrombosis of Prosthetic Heart Valves: Recommendations

Class I

1. Transthoracic and Doppler echocardiography is indicated in patients with suspected prosthetic valve thrombosis to assess hemodynamic severity. *(Level of Evidence: B)*
2. Transesophageal echocardiography and/or fluoroscopy is indicated in patients with suspected valve thrombosis to assess valve motion and clot burden. *(Level of Evidence: B)*

Class IIa

1. Emergency operation is reasonable for patients with a thrombosed left-sided prosthetic valve and NYHA functional class III–IV symptoms. *(Level of Evidence: C)*
2. Emergency operation is reasonable for patients with a thrombosed left-sided prosthetic valve and a large clot burden. *(Level of Evidence: C)*
3. Fibrinolytic therapy is reasonable for thrombosed right-sided prosthetic heart valves with NYHA class III–IV symptoms or a large clot burden. *(Level of Evidence C)*

Class IIb

1. Fibrinolytic therapy may be considered as a first-line therapy for patients with a thrombosed left-sided prosthetic valve, NYHA functional class I–II symptoms, and a small clot burden. *(Level of Evidence: B)*
2. Fibrinolytic therapy may be considered as a first-line therapy for patients with a thrombosed left-sided prosthetic valve, NYHA functional class III–IV symptoms, and a small clot burden if surgery is high risk or not available. *(Level of Evidence: B)*

3. Fibrinolytic therapy may be considered for patients with an obstructed, thrombosed left-sided prosthetic valve who have NYHA functional class II–IV symptoms and a large clot burden if emergency surgery is high risk or not available. *(Level of Evidence: C)*

4. Intravenous UFH as an alternative to fibrinolytic therapy may be considered for patients with a thrombosed valve who are in NYHA functional class I–II and have a small clot burden. *(Level of Evidence: C)*

Prosthetic valve endocarditis (PVE)

Definition: Prosthetic valvular endocarditis is any infection involving an operated valve

Early PVE:

   Within 60 days of valve replacement surgery

   Incidence: 2 %

   Source of infection:

      Surgical contamination

      Immediate post operative infection

   Organisms:

      Staphylococcus aureas

      Staphylococcus epidemidis

      Rarely: Gram negative bacteria or fungus

   Poor response to medical therapy

   High mortality rate; > 50 %

Late PVE:

   After 60 days of valve surgery

   Incidence: 1 -2 % / yr (According to Braunwald 0.2 – 0.35 % per year)

   Mimics sub acute bacterial endocarditis

Organisms:
- Streptococci
- Rarely
  - Staphylococci
  - Gram negative bacteria
  - Fungus

Better response to medical therapy as compared to early PVE
- Mortality: 25 %
- Reasons:
  - Less virulent organisms
  - More sensitive to antibiotics
  - Medical Rx is more effective if there are no new regurgitant murmurs

Surgery for Prosthetic Valve Endocarditis: Recommendations

Class I

1. Consultation with a cardiac surgeon is indicated for patients with infective endocarditis of a prosthetic valve. *(Level of Evidence: C)*

2. Surgery is indicated for patients with infective endocarditis of a prosthetic valve who present with heart failure. *(Level of Evidence: B)*

3. Surgery is indicated for patients with infective endocarditis of a prosthetic valve who present with dehiscence evidenced by cine fluoroscopy or echocardiography. *(Level of Evidence: B)*

4. Surgery is indicated for patients with infective endocarditis of a prosthetic valve who present with evidence of increasing obstruction or worsening regurgitation. *(Level of Evidence: C)*

5. Surgery is indicated for patients with infective endocarditis of a prosthetic valve who present with complications, for example, abscess formation. *(Level of Evidence: C)*

Class IIa

1. Surgery is reasonable for patients with infective endocarditis of a prosthetic valve who present with evidence of persistent bacteremia or recurrent emboli despite appropriate antibiotic treatment. *(Level of Evidence: C)*
2. Surgery is reasonable for patients with infective endocarditis of a prosthetic valve who present with relapsing infection. *(Level of Evidence: C)*

Class III

Routine surgery is not indicated for patients with uncomplicated infective endocarditis of a prosthetic valve caused by first infection with a sensitive organism. *(Level of Evidence: C)*

Hemolysis

More common with prosthetic valve in aortic position (* valve thrombosis more common in mitral position)
Caged ball more likely to cause hemolysis than disc valves
Caged ball > Disc valves > Bioprosthetic valves
Highest incidence in noncloth covered Starr-Edwards aortic valve

Reasons:
>   If blood flows through stenotic orifices like stenotic valves or slitlike perivalvular leaks, hemolysis is common
>   Coexisting anemia can worsen this factor
>   Valvar or paravalvar leaks striking on cardiac walls
>   For these 2 reasons, bioprosthetic valves can cause as severe hemolysis as mechanical valves
>   Less central and more turbulent flow (more with caged ball)
>   Red cell compression (more with caged ball)
>   Increased fragility of RBC; iron deficiency, fragmented RBCs

Diagnosis of hemolysis:
>   RBC morphology
>> Schistocytosis
>> Reticulocytosis
>   Hemosidenuria
>   Absent serum haptoglobin

Increased serum LDH

Management:

Iron and folate supplements

Blood transfusions if serious

* Replacement of valve is indicated only if anemia is refractory to treatment and causes high output failure or is due to significant valve dysfunction.

Structural Failure of Prosthetic Valves

Should be suspected if a patient with prosthesis develops
  Progressive or rapidly worsening dyspnea
  Syncope or presyncope
  New or worsening of angina
  Increasing hemolysis
  Transient ischemic attacks

Caged ball valves:
  Strut failure
      Strut failure   0.087 % / yr (Bjork Shiley)
  Ball variance (rare)
  Sewing ring dehiscence

Disc valve
  Sewing ring dehiscence; secondary to PVE
  Thrombosis interfering with proper disc motion
  Eccentric wearing of disc

Bioprosthesis
  Spontaneous tissue degeneration
  Leaflet perforation
  Leaflet calcification (may cause stenosis or regurgitation)

Ball variance:

Valve malfunction due to chemical or physical alteration of the occluder

Results in swelling, fissuring, fracture, or fragmentation and formation of fluid lakes in the core of the occluder

May lead to impaction, dislodgement or embolization

Rare in currently used caged ball valves

Disc valves have a very low rate of mechanical or structural failure but are prone to thrombotic occlusion. This may cause disc immobility (reduced opening angle) with obstruction and severe regurgitation.

Disc variance:

Disc moves up and down in a fixed axis. This movement results in an uneven distribution of stress on contracting parts. If the disc wears to an extent that it cannot cover the primary orifice, prosthetic regurgitation results.

Impact wear and friction wear dictate the loss of material in prosthetic valve. Impact wear usually occurs in the hinge regions of bileaflets, between the occluder and ring in tilting-discs, and between the ball and cage in caged-ball valves. Friction wear occurs between the occluder and strut in tilting-discs, and between the leaflet pivots and hinge cavities in bileaflets

Cavitation

Cavitation is an event that can lead to prosthesis failure. Cavitation is the rapid formation of vaporous microbubbles in the fluid due to a local drop of pressure below the vaporization pressure at a given temperature. When conditions for cavitation are present bubbles will form and at the time of pressure recovery they will collapse or implode. This event will cause pressure or thermal shockwaves and fluid microjets which can damage a surface. These thermodynamic conditions are known to be the cause of prosthesis related erosion.

The valvular event that causes such cavitating conditions to exist is the closing mechanics of the prosthesis. Several causes of cavitation relating to valve closure have been identified. Squeeze flow is the term used to describe cavitation that is said to occur as the occluder approaches the housing during closure and fluid is squeezed between the occluder and the valve housing causing a low pressure formation. Water hammer is a term used to describe cavitation caused by the sudden stop of the valve occluder as it contacts the valve housing. This sudden retard of the fluid retrograde inertia is said to put the fluid under tension causing cavitation. Squeeze flow is said to form a cloud of bubbles at the circumferential lip of the occluder whereas water hammer is said to be seen as transient bubbles at the occlude housing.

For either event, cavitation occurs on the upstream side of valve. Clinically, cavitation is of primary concern in the mitral position. This position is especially harsh due to the sudden ventricular pressure rise which drives the valve closure against a low left atrial pressure which is said to be the worst case condition thus position for cavitation to occur. Cavitation is also suspected as a contributing factor in blood cell damage and increased risk of thromboembloic complications.

The temporal rate of change of the left ventricular, measured as a slope of the ventricular pressure curve (dP/dt) is regarded as the best indicator for cavitation potential.

Tissue valve: Structural failure

Age of patient	Duration of valve replacement	Failure rate
> 65 yrs		Extremely low
> 35 yrs		
	First 7 yrs	1-2 % / yr
	10 yrs	25 %
	15 yrs	65 %
< 35 yrs		
	At 10 yrs	50 %
< 30 yrs		
	At 10 yrs	75 %
< 20 yrs		
	At 6 yrs	80 %

Homograft valve

	Reoperation free interval
At 10 yrs	90 %
At 19 yrs	50 %

Causes of left ventricular failure in patients with valve replacement
    Structural failure of valve
    Endocarditis
    Chronic myocardial dysfunction due to valve disease
    Associated CAD

Patient prosthesis mismatch (PPM)

Term proposed by Rahimtoola in 1978

Cause of *Nonstructural dysfunction* of the valve

Results due to 'Inappropriate sizing' of the prosthesis

 A normally functioning prosthesis is too small in relation to the patient's body size (and therefore cardiac output requirements), resulting in abnormally high postoperative gradients

 Individuals in whom a small prosthetic valve is implanted due to small aortic or mitral annulus

Clinical Impact of PPM

 Less improvement in symptoms and functional class

 Impaired exercise capacity

 More adverse cardiac events

 Less regression of LVH (Aortic PPM)

 Less improvement in coronary flow reserve (Aortic PPM)

 Impact is more significant in patients with depressed LV function and has increased post operative mortality

 Impact of PPM also is more pronounced in young patients than in older patients, which might be related to the fact that younger patients have higher cardiac output requirements and are exposed to the risk of PPM for a longer period of time.

Prevention of PPM

 Aortic PPM

 Avoided by systematically calculating the projected indexed effective orifice area (EOA) of the prosthesis to be inserted

 If PPM is anticipated then, by using alternate procedures such as insertion of a prosthesis model with better hemodynamic performance and aortic root enlargement to accommodate a larger size of the same prosthesis model

 Mitral PPM

 A greater challenge than in the aortic position because valve annulus enlargement or stentless valve implantation is not an option in this situation

Prosthetic valve evaluation: Echocardiography

Echocardiography has greatly simplified the follow up of prosthetic valves

Evaluation and interpretation should be done in light of type of valve used for replacement. The design of valve and its occluder affect the range of transvalvular velocities and gradients and there is considerable overlap in normal values of different valve types and size. (See hemodynamics of prosthetic valves).

All prosthetic valves are inherently obstructive and have their own regurgitant patterns. The Echo-Doppler study must be done in for each valve in the early post operative period for subsequent follow up reference.

Evaluation should be done by transthoracic method and if required by transesophageal method if valve dysfunction is suspected.

Parameters to be measured:
    Basics:
        Dimensions of all cardiac chambers
        LV function
        Analysis of other (normal) valves
        Pulmonary hypertension estimation
    Prosthetic evaluation
    Prosthesis
        Identification of sewing ring, occluder mechanism and surrounding area
        Evaluation of disc or leaflet excursion
            Transvalvular gradients
            Effective valve area
            Prosthetic regurgitation
                Physiological
                Pathological
    Identification of prosthesis mechanism:
        Helps to distinguish patient-prosthesis mismatch with valve dysfunction
        Disc or leaflet excursion is an important point in identify-

ing valve thrombosis or pannus (on Echo, differentiation between thrombus and pannus may be difficult)

Transvalvular gradients:

All prosthesis are inherently stenotic and hence some gradients are always expected. Prosthetic stenosis is usually implied if the peak velocity is > 2.5 m / sec across mitral prosthesis (25 mm Hg) and > 4m/sec across aortic prosthesis (64 mm Hg).

Interpretation of High Gradients: Distinguishing Between High-Flow States, PPM, and Pathological Valve Obstruction

Diagnosis of increased transprosthetic gradient

Mean gradient

>15 to 20 mm Hg for aortic prostheses and

>5 to 7 mm Hg for mitral prostheses

A high gradient can be due to

An associated subvalvular obstruction or

A high-flow state (e.g., hyperadrenergism, valvular regurgitation); such occurrences can be suspected when the Doppler velocity index (DVI) is normal (>0.35 for aortic or >0.45 for mitral prostheses).

Combination of a high gradient and a low DVI

Suggests valvular obstruction

In such cases, an integrative evaluation must be done; in particular, the distinction must be made between obstruction resulting from PPM, which is by far the most frequent cause of high postoperative gradients, and intrinsic prosthesis dysfunction, which is a pathological condition requiring more investigation and treatment.

Effective valve area:

Gorlin formula:

Several limitations

Tends to underestimate prosthetic orifice area under conditions of low pressure gradient or flow and overestimate in opposite conditions.

Pressure half time

Mainly used for mitral prosthesis

Easy to calculate

Not a reliable method

Factors affecting PHT are heart rate, diastolic filling period, stroke volume, ventricular compliance and pressure gradients at the start of diastole

Continuity equation

More accurate than other methods

Cumbersome and time consuming

Small errors in measurement can lead to wide fluctuation in area

Other parameters:

Performance index:

Defined as the effective orifice area divided by the calculated primary orifice area

Primary orifice area is the calculated area as defined as determined from the orifice diameter without the occluder

It has significant but inverse correlation between valve size and performance index

Doppler velocity index (DVI):

Ratio of blood velocity in the left ventricular outflow to across the prosthesis

Mainly depends on flow and much less on valve size

DVI is always less than unity and a value less than 0.27 raises the suspicion of significant valve obstruction Normal value: >0.35 for aortic or >0.45 for mitral prostheses.

Valve resistance:

Valve resistance = (MPG x ET / SV) x 1.33 in dyne. sec. cm^{-5}

Where MPG: Mean prosthetic gradient in mm Hg

ET: Ejection time in seconds

SV: Stroke volume in ml/min

Limited data for various valves

For ST. Jude aortic prosthesis the normal value is 85 +/- 38

Prosthetic Aortic Valve Stenosis: Echocardiographic Assessment

A) Effective AVA

Effective AVA = SV / TVI jet

= CSA lvo X TVI lvo / TVI jet

Where

Effective AVA in sq. cm

SV: Stroke volume in ml

TVI jet: Time velocity integral of aortic jet in cm

TVI lvo: Time velocity integral LVO in cm

CSA lvo: Cross-sectional area of LVO in sq. cm

lvo / LVO; Left ventricular outflow

B) Doppler Velocity Index (DVI)

DVI = VELOCITY lvo / VELOCITY jet

= Peak VELOCITY lvo / Peak VELOCITY jet

Where

VELOCITY jet: velocity of aortic jet in cm

VELOCITY lvo: velocity LVO in cm

lvo / LVO; Left ventricular outflow

C)   Valve Resistance

Valve resistance = (MPG x ET / SV) x 1.33 in dyne.sec. cm^{-5}

   Where MPG: Mean prosthetic gradient in mm Hg

   ET: Ejection time in seconds

   SV: Stroke volume in ml/min

Prosthetic Mitral Valve Stenosis: Echocardiographic Assessment

A)   Effective MVA

Effective MVA = SV / TVI mvjet

   Where

   Effective MVA in sq. cm

   SV: Stroke volume in ml

   TVI mvjet: Time velocity integral of MV jet in cm

B)   Pressure Half Time (PHT)

Effective MVA = 220 / PHT

   Concept same as native valve

Prosthetic regurgitation: Echocardiographic assessment

Important to identify physiological regurgitation patterns

2 patterns of physiologic regurgitation have been seen:

Dynamic regurgitation or closure back flow i.e., blood volume necessary to close the occluder

Static regurgitation or leakage backflow i.e., blood volume passing the occluder and housing during diastole at aortic and in systole at mitral position

It is shown that some regurgitation occurs in all types of prosthesis ranging from 0.2 % to 30 % of the forward flow, but rarely exceeding 10 %.

Theoretically it is possible to detect regurgitant flow in all prosthesis.

Physiological regurgitation:

Physiological regurgitation is characterized by its early onset, short duration, narrow width, low velocity (absence of flow convergence) and a homogenous color (red or blue). It reflects backflow from the closing movement of ball or disc(s). In contrast pathological regurgitant jets are longer in duration; wide, asymmetrical across the valve midline, frequently eccentric and display a mosaic pattern reflecting high velocity turbulent flow.

Transesophageal echocardiography (TEE) is much better in assessing the severity and distinguishing between physiological and pathological regurgitation.

Bioprosthetic and Medtronic Hall valves have single central jet, tilting disc prosthesis have 2 jets and bileaflet prosthesis have 3 jets of forward flow. It has been shown that a regurgitant jet area of less than 2 cm^2 and jet length of less than 2.5 cm in mitral position, and a jet area of less than 1 cm^2 and jet length of less than 1.5 cm in the aortic position are normal findings on TEE examination.

Tilting disc and bileaflet valves have built-in, additional leakage backflow occurring later, when the prosthesis is fully closed. The purpose of this design is to reduce the risk of valve thrombosis.

Paraprosthetic regurgitation:

Always pathological

Paraprosthetic regurgitation should always be taken seriously and even trivial regurgitation should be followed up regularly.

Prosthetic Aortic Valve regurgitation: Echocardiographic assessment

Criteria for grading severity are similar to those of native aortic valve

Moderately severe or worse regurgitation is diagnosed in presence of at least 2 of the following

1) Jet width more than 50% of left ventricular outflow diameter
2) A dense, holodiastolic regurgitant jet, with PHT less than 350 ms
3) Holodiastolic flow reversal in descending aorta

4) Regurgitant fraction more than 40%

Prosthetic Mitral Valve regurgitation: Echocardiographic assessment
Significant mitral prosthetic regurgitation is suggested by
1) Signs of increased mitral inflow volume (peak early velocity more than 1.9 m/s without signs of obstruction, i.e., PHT less than 120 ms)
2) Decreased systemic output despite normal left ventricular function, with ratio of left ventricular outflow time velocity integral of mitral inflow 0.4 or less.
3) Short isovolumic relaxation time (less than 70 ms)
4) Dense regurgitant jet by CW Doppler, with early maximal velocity.
5) Regurgitant fraction more than 50%
6) Flow convergence proximal isovelocity surface area (PISA) on the ventricular side of the valve
7) Unexplained pulmonary hypertension

Valve thrombosis: Echocardiography

Valve thrombosis: Progressive increase in transprosthetic gradients could be due to pannus formation or valve thrombosis. The echocardiographic distinction between two may be extremely difficult. Valve thrombosis may lead to rapid worsening or symptoms.

As in all valve complications, TEE is a much better modality to identify thrombosis.

PVE (Prosthetic Valve Endocarditis) on echocardiography:
Manifestations of PVE include:

Irregular, frequently mobile, masses attached to valves or cardiac walls (jet lesions)

Interference with occluder function: Resulting in stenosis and / or regurgitation

Leaflet destruction (Bioprosthesis)

Perivalvular abscess

Prosthesis rocking

Periprosthetic thickening

Periprosthetic echolucency

TEE is far superior to TTE in detection of vegetations. If negative on first examination and there is strong clinical suspicion of PVE, TEE should be repeated after 15 days to increase chances of finding vegetations.

Stress echocardiography:
A useful investigation to evaluate patients of prosthetic valves, who have normal resting echocardiographic data but are symptomatic.

Antithrombotic Therapy after prosthetic valve surgery

Class I

1. After AVR with bileaflet mechanical or Medtronic Hall prostheses, in patients with no risk factors,* warfarin is indicated to achieve an INR of 2.0 to 3.0. If the patient has risk factors, warfarin is indicated to achieve an INR of 2.5 to 3.5. *(Level of Evidence: B)*

2. After AVR with Starr-Edwards valves or mechanical disc valves (other than Medtronic Hall prostheses), in patients with no risk factors,* warfarin is indicated to achieve an INR of 2.5 to 3.5. *(Level of Evidence: B)*

3. After MV replacement with any mechanical valve, warfarin is indicated to achieve an INR of 2.5 to 3.5. *(Level of Evidence: C)*

4. After AVR or MV replacement with a bioprosthesis and no risk factors,* aspirin is indicated at 75 to 100 mg per day. *(Level of Evidence: C)*

5. After AVR with a bioprosthesis and risk factors,* warfarin is indicated to achieve an INR of 2.0 to 3.0. *(Level of Evidence: C)*

6. After MV replacement with a bioprosthesis and risk factors,* warfarin is indicated to achieve an INR of 2.0 to 3.0. *(Level of Evidence: C)*

7. For those patients who are unable to take warfarin after MV replacement or AVR, aspirin is indicated in a dose of 75 to 325 mg per day. *(Level of Evidence: B)*

8. The addition of aspirin 75 to 100 mg once daily to therapeutic warfarin is recommended for all patients with mechanical heart valves and those patients with biological valves who have risk factors.* *(Level of Evidence: B)*

Class IIa

1. During the first 3 months after AVR with a mechanical prosthesis, it is reasonable to give warfarin to achieve an INR of 2.5 to 3.5. *(Level of Evidence: C)*

2. During the first 3 months after AVR or MV replacement with a bioprosthesis, in patients with no risk factors,* it is reasonable to give warfarin to achieve an INR of 2.0 to 3.0. *(Level of Evidence: C)*

Class IIb

In high-risk patients with prosthetic heart valves in whom aspirin cannot be used, it may be reasonable to give clopidogrel (75 mg per day) or warfarin to achieve an INR of 3.5 to 4.5. *(Level of Evidence: C)*

*Risk factors include atrial fibrillation, previous thromboembolism, LV dysfunction, and hypercoagulable condition.

Depending on patients' clinical status, antithrombotic therapy must be individualized. In patients receiving warfarin, aspirin is recommended in virtually all situations. Risk factors: atrial fibrillation, left ventricular dysfunction, previous thromboembolism, and hypercoagulable condition. International normalized ratio (INR) should be maintained between 2.5 and 3.5 for aortic disc valves and Starr-Edwards valves. Modified from McAnulty JH, Rahimtoola SH. Antithrombotic therapy in valvular heart disease. In:Schlant R, Alexander RW, editors. Hurst's The Heart. New York, NY: McGraw-Hill, 1998:1867–74 (934).

Anticoagulation regimen after prosthetic valve surgery: Summary

	Warfarin (INR 2 – 3)	Warfarin (INR 2.5 – 3.5)	Aspirin
Mechanical prosthetic valves			
First 3 months post surgery		+	+
After first 3 months of surgery			
Aortic valve†	+		+
Aortic valve and risk factors		+	+
Mitral valve		+	+
Mitral valve and risk factors		+	+
Bioprosthetic valves			
First 3 months post surgery		+	+
After first 3 months of surgery			
Aortic valve			+
Aortic valve and risk factors	+		+
Mitral valve			+
Mitral valve and risk factors		+	+

Aspirin should be given in 80 – 100 mg doses

Risk factors: Atrial fibrillation, LV dysfunction, previous thromboembolism, and hypercoagulable condition.

†INR should be maintained between 2.5 and 3.5 for aortic disc valves and Starr- Edwards valves.

+: Recommended regimen

Pregnancy and Prosthetic Valves

Management of prosthetic valve anticoagulation in pregnancy

Pregnancy is associated with an increased risk of prosthetic valve related morbidity and mortality. Fetal loss is higher with warfarin based regimens and maternal loss is higher with heparin based regimens. Anticoagulation presents a separate management problem during pregnancy. The physiological changes in cardiovascular system may lead to worsening of cardiac symptoms during pregnancy. Moreover, pregnancy is considered to be hypercoagulable state and there is significant inter-individual variability. Thus the degree to which any woman is hypercoagulable is unpredictable.

Anticoagulation regimens proposed during pregnancy:
    Warfarin based regimen
    Heparin based regimen
    Mixed regimens

Issues related to warfarin use during pregnancy

    Warfarin syndrome:
        Warfarin crosses placenta and is associated with early and late teratogenic effects. The majority of these effects are the result of fetal exposure between 6th and 12th weeks of pregnancy.
    'Classical' warfarin embryopathy: Fetal abnormalities ranging from
        Nasal hypoplasia
        Stippled epiphyses (Chondrodysplasia)
        CNS abnormalities and other malformations
    Outside the 'Classical' features, others (common) include:
        Fetal wastage
        Scarring as a result of fetal hemorrhage
        Mental retardation
        Blindness and other CNS abnormalities
        Congenital heart disease

Polydactyly
Other malformations

Incidence of Warfarin syndrome:
Very variable reports in literature (4 – 67 %). Recent larger studies suggest the incidence to be around 4 – 10 %. After 12th week of gestation the risk is less than 5 %.
Warfarin syndrome risk appears to be **dose dependent**. Woman requiring more than 5 mg of Warfarin per day is at substantially higher risk.

Issues related to heparin in pregnancy:
Heparin related side effects:
Maternal hemorrhage
Osteopenia
Thrombocytopenia
Fetal loss secondary to retro placental hemorrhage
Advantage: No direct teratogenic effects (does not cross placenta)
Dose: Dose to keep aPTT 2-3 times control, measured 6 hours after dosing. aPTT levels should be monitored (6 hour troughs) daily during initiation of treatment and a minimum of twice weekly thereafter (bioavailability of UFH is less consistent than LMWH)

Thromboembolic rate for mechanical prosthesis during pregnancy
On IV heparin regimen
8 – 29 %
On subcutaneous UFH regimen
12 – 24 %
Role of LMWH (Low molecular weight heparin)
No definite recommendations to be used as a substitute to UFH in pregnancy with mechanical prosthesis
If used, it is advisable to monitor peak and 4 hour trough anti Factor Xa levels at least every few days on initiation

and a minimum of weekly thereafter in anticipation of weight gain and alteration in body fluid composition.

Dose: 1 mg/ kg of Enoxaparin SC BID

Recommended 4 hour trough anti Factor Xa levels: 0.5 – 1.1 IU/ml

Recommendations for anticoagulation during pregnancy in patients with mechanical prosthesis.

Weeks 1 - 35

Class I indications:

The decision whether to use heparin during the first trimester or to continue oral anticoagulation throughout the pregnancy should be made after full discussion with the patient and her partner (husband); if she chooses to change to heparin for the first trimester, she should be made aware that heparin is less safe for her, with a higher risk of both thrombosis and bleeding and that any risk to her also jeopardizes the baby.

High risk women (history of thromboembolism or an older generation mechanical prosthesis in mitral position) who choose not to take warfarin during the first trimester should receive continuous unfractionated heparin (UFH) IV in a dose to prolong the midinterval (6 hours after dosing) aPTT to 2-3 times control. Transition to warfarin can occur thereafter.

Class IIa indication:

In patients receiving warfarin, INR should be maintained between 2 – 3 with the lowest possible dose of warfarin, and low dose aspirin should be added.

Class IIb indication:

Women at lower risk (no history of thromboembolism,

newer low profile prosthesis) may be managed with adjusted-dose subcutaneous UFH (17,500 – 20,000 IU BID) to prolong midinterval (6 hours after dosing) aPTT to 2-3 times control.

A possible clinical approach to anticoagulation in pregnancy

Step I:

Evaluate patient and husband's wishes in regards to the importance of the safety of the patient versus safety of the baby.

If 'safety of the patient' is the choice:
Step II:

Evaluate risk associated with valve type, position and other co morbidities such as AF, previous thromboembolism, ventricular dysfunction, multiple valves)

High risk valve: (Presence of any of these risk factors)
1 Strongly consider warfarin throughout the pregnancy until 36 weeks
2 At week 36 switch to IV UFH in a dose to prolong the midinterval (6 hours after dosing) aPTT to 2-3 times control.
3 Strongly consider low dose aspirin throughout pregnancy

Low risk valve:
1. Recommend warfarin till 36 weeks of pregnancy. IV or SC UFH can be used during 6 to 12 weeks of gestation.
2. At week 36 switch to IV UFH in a dose to prolong the midinterval (6 hours after dosing) aPTT to 2-3 times control.
3. Strongly consider low dose aspirin throughout pregnancy

If 'safety of the fetus' is the choice
Step II:
Evaluate risk associated with valve type, position and other comorbidities such as AF, previous thromboembolism, ventricular dysfunction, multiple valves)

High risk valve: (Presence of any of these risk factors)
1. Favor IV UFH throughout pregnancy, although could consider warfarin with UFH substitution weeks 6 – 12 and after 36 weeks, particularly if maternal warfarin requirement is low (< 5 mg/day)
2. Strongly consider low dose aspirin throughout pregnancy

Low risk valve:
1. Consider adjusted dose SC UFH (17,500 – 20,000 IU BID) to prolong midinterval (6 hours after dosing) aPTT to 2-3 times control, throughout the pregnancy
2. Strongly consider low dose aspirin throughout pregnancy

Selection of Anticoagulation Regimen in Pregnant Patients with Mechanical Prosthetic Valves

Class I

1. All pregnant patients with mechanical prosthetic valves must receive continuous therapeutic anticoagulation with frequent monitoring (see Section 9.2 of the original guideline document). *(Level of Evidence: B)*

2. For women requiring long-term warfarin therapy who are attempting pregnancy, pregnancy tests should be monitored with discussions about subsequent anticoagulation therapy, so that anticoagulation can be continued uninterrupted when pregnancy is achieved. *(Level of Evidence: C)*

3. Pregnant patients with mechanical prosthetic valves who elect to stop warfarin between weeks 6 and 12 of gestation should receive

continuous intravenous unfractionated heparin (UFH), dose-adjusted UFH, or dose-adjusted subcutaneous low molecular weight heparin (LMWH). *(Level of Evidence: C)*

4. For pregnant patients with mechanical prosthetic valves, up to 36 weeks of gestation, the therapeutic choice of continuous intravenous or dose-adjusted subcutaneous UFH, dose-adjusted LMWH, or warfarin should be discussed fully. If continuous intravenous UFH is used, the fetal risk is lower, but the maternal risks of prosthetic valve thrombosis, systemic embolization, infection, osteoporosis, and heparin-induced thrombocytopenia are relatively higher. *(Level of Evidence: C)*

5. In pregnant patients with mechanical prosthetic valves who receive dose-adjusted LMWH, the LMWH should be administered twice daily subcutaneously to maintain the anti-Xa level between 0.7 and 1.2 units (U) per ml 4 h after administration. *(Level of Evidence: C)*

6. In pregnant patients with mechanical prosthetic valves who receive dose-adjusted UFH, the activated partial thromboplastin time (aPTT) should be at least twice control. *(Level of Evidence: C)*

7. In pregnant patients with mechanical prosthetic valves who receive warfarin, the international normalized ratio (INR) goal should be 3.0 (range 2.5 to 3.5). *(Level of Evidence: C)*

8. In pregnant patients with mechanical prosthetic valves, warfarin should be discontinued and continuous intravenous UFH given starting 2 to 3 weeks before planned delivery. *(Level of Evidence: C)*

Class IIa

1. In patients with mechanical prosthetic valves, it is reasonable to avoid warfarin between weeks 6 and 12 of gestation owing to the high risk of fetal defects. (Level of Evidence: C)

2. In patients with mechanical prosthetic valves, it is reasonable to resume UFH 4 to 6 h after delivery and begin oral warfarin in the absence of significant bleeding. (Level of Evidence: C)

3. In patients with mechanical prosthetic valves, it is reasonable to give low-dose aspirin (75 to 100 mg per day) in the second and third trimesters of pregnancy in addition to anticoagulation with warfarin or heparin. (Level of Evidence: C)

Class III
1. LMWH should not be administered to pregnant patients with mechanical prosthetic valves unless anti-Xa levels are monitored 4 to 6 h after administration. (Level of Evidence: C)

2. Dipyridamole should not be used instead of aspirin as an alternative antiplatelet agent in pregnant patients with mechanical prosthetic valves because of its harmful effects on the fetus. (Level *of Evidence: B)*

Management of Prosthetic valve thrombosis during pregnancy

Options:

Surgery:

Indications:

High thrombus burden

NYHA class $\geq$ III

Evidence of severe valve obstruction

Maternal mortality: 6 %

Maternal morbidity: 24 %

Fetal mortality: 30 %

Thrombolytic Therapy:

Can be used

Disadvantage:

Ineffective or incomplete thrombolysis especially in cases of large thrombus burden

Major bleeding: 5 %

Cerebrovascular accident: 3 – 10 %

Maternal mortality: 1.2 %

Pregnancy loss rate: 6 %

Antibiotics Prophylaxis for Infective Endocarditis

Regimens for Dental, Oral, Respiratory Tract, or Esophageal Procedures

Situation	Agent	Regimen*
Standard general prophylaxis		
	Amoxicillin	Adults: 2.0 g; Children: 50 mg/kg PO 1 h before procedure.
Unable to take oral medication		
	Ampicillin	Adults: 2.0 g IM or IV; Children: 50 mg/kg IM or IV within 30 min before procedure.
Penicillin-allergic		
	Clindamycin or	Adults: 600 mg; Children: 20 mg/kg PO 1 h before procedure.
	Cephalexin† or cephadroxil†	Adults: 2.0 g; Children 50 mg/kg PO 1 h before procedure.
	Or Azithromycin or clarithromycin	Adults: 500 mg; Children 15 mg/kg PO 1 h before procedure.
Penicillin-allergic & unable to take oral medications		
	Clindamycin or	Adults: 600 mg; Children 20 mg/kg IV within 30 min before procedure.
	Cefazolin†	Adults: 1.0 g; Children: 25 mg/kg IM or IV within min before procedure.

*Total children's dose should not exceed adult dose.
†Cephalosporins should not be used in individuals with immediate-type hypersensitivity reaction (urticaria, angioedema, or anaphylaxis) to penicillins.

Regimens for Genitourinary/Gastrointestinal (Excluding Esophageal) Procedures

Patients with prosthetic valves come under 'high risk' category prophylaxis.

Situation	Agent(s)*	Regimen†
High-risk patients		
	Ampicillin plus gentamicin	
		Adults:
		Ampicillin: 2.0 g IM/IV plus Gentamicin: 1.5 mg/kg (not to exceed 120 mg) within 30 min of starting the procedure.
		Six hours later:
		Ampicillin: 1 g IM/IV or amoxicillin 1 g PO.
		Children:
		Ampicillin: 50 mg/kg IM or IV (not to exceed 2.0 g) plus Gentamicin: 1.5 mg/kg within 30 min of starting the procedure.
		Six hours later:
		Ampicillin: 25 mg/kg IM/IV or amoxicillin: 25 mg/kg PO.
High-risk patients allergic to ampicillin/amoxicillin		
	Vancomycin plus gentamicin	
		Adults:
		Vancomycin: 1.0 g IV over 1–2 h plus Gentamicin: 1.5 mg/kg IV/IM (not to exceed 120 mg). Complete injection/infusion within 30 min of starting the procedure.
		Children:
		Vancomycin: 20 mg/kg IV over 1–2 h plus Gentamicin: 1.5 mg/kg IV/IM. Complete injection/infusion within 30 min of starting the procedure.

*No second dose of vancomycin or gentamicin is recommended.
†Total children's dose should not exceed adult dose.

Suggested Reading

1. Bonow RO, Carabello BA, Kanu C, *et al.* (2006). "ACC/AHA 2006 guidelines for the management of patients with valvular heart disease: a report of the American College of Cardiology/American Heart Association Task Force on Practice Guidelines (writing committee to revise the 1998 Guidelines for the Management of Patients With Valvular Heart Disease): developed in collaboration with the Society of Cardiovascular Anesthesiologists: endorsed by the Society for Cardiovascular Angiography and Interventions and the Society of Thoracic Surgeons". *Circulation* **114** (5): e84–231

2. Vahanian A, Baumgartner H, Bax J, Butchart E, Dion R, Filippatos G, Flachskampf F, Hall R, Iung B, Kasprzak J, Nataf P, Tornos P, Torracca L, Wenink A. Guidelines on the management of valvular heart disease: the Task Force on the Management of Valvular Heart Disease of the European Society of Cardiology. Eur Heart J. 2007; 28: 230–268

3. Elkayam U, Bitar F. Valvular heart disease and pregnancy, part II: prosthetic valves. J Am Coll Cardiol. 2005; 46: 403–410

4. Butchart EG, Gohlke-Barwolf C, Antunes MJ, Tornos P, De Caterina R, Cormier B, Prendergast B, Iung B, Bjornstad H, Leport C, Hall RJ, Vahanian A, for the Working Groups on Valvular Heart Disease, Thrombosis, and Cardiac Rehabilitation and Exercise Physiology, European Society of Cardiology. Recommendations for the management of patients after heart valve surgery. Eur Heart J. 2005; 26: 2463–2471

5. Jamieson WR, Cartier PC, Allard M, Boutin C, Burwash IG, Butany J, de Varennes B, Del Rizzo D, Dumesnil JG, Honos G, Houde C, Munt BI, Poirier N, Rebeyka IM, Ross DB, Siu SC, Williams WG, Rebeyka IM, David TE, Dyck JD, Feindel CM, Fradet GJ, Human DG, Lemieux MD, Menkis AH, Scully HE, Turpie AG, Adams DH, Berrebi A, Chambers J, Chang KL, Cohn LH, Duran CM, Elkins RC, Freedman R, Huysman HA, Jue J, Perier P, Rakowski H, Schaff HV, Schoen FA, Shah P, Thompson CR, Warnes C, Westaby S, Yacoub MH. Surgical management of

valvular heart disease 2004. Can J Cardiol. 2004; 20 (suppl E): 7E–120E

6. McAnulty JH, Rahimtoola SH. Antithrombotic therapy for valvular heart disease. In: Fuster V, O'Rourke RA, Walsh RA, Poole-Wilson P, eds. Hurst's The Heart. New York, NY: McGraw-Hill; 2008: 1800–1807

7. Vesey JM, Otto CM. Complications of prosthetic heart valves. Curr Cardiol Rep. 2004; 6: 106–111.

8. Horstkotte D, Follath F, Gutschik E, Lengyel M, Oto A, Pavie A, Soler-Soler J, Thiene G, von Graevenitz A, Priori SG, Garcia MA, Blanc JJ, Budaj A, Cowie M, Dean V, Deckers J, Fernández Burgos E, Lekakis J, Lindahl B, Mazzotta G, Morais J, Oto A, Smiseth OA, Lekakis J, Vahanian A, Delahaye F, Parkhomenko A, Filipatos G, Aldershvile J, Vardas P, for the Task Force Members on Infective Endocarditis of the European Society of Cardiology, ESC Committee for Practice Guidelines (CPG), Document Reviewers. Guidelines on prevention, diagnosis and treatment of infective endocarditis executive summary: the Task Force on Infective Endocarditis of the European Society of Cardiology. Eur Heart J. 2004; 25: 267–276

9. Deloche A, Guerinon J, Fabiani JN, et al. Anatomical study of rheumatic tricuspid valve diseases: application to the study of various valvuloplasties. Ann Chir Thorac Cardiovasc 1973;12:343–9.

10. Rapaport E: Calculation of valve areas. Eur Heart J 1985; 6 (suppl C): 21.

11. Chapter 66: Valvular Heart Disease. Braunwald's Heart Disease(Elsevier), 9th ed., 1468-1539.

12. Chapters 11: Combined Valvular Disease. Valvular Heart Disease. Edited by Dalen and Alpert (Little, brown and company). 2th ed., 439-508.

13. Chapters 12: Prosthetic Heart Valves. Valvular Heart Disease.

Edited by Dalen and Alpert (Little, brown and company). 2th ed., 509-528.

14. Rahimtoola SH. Perspective on valvular heart disease : Update II. In : Knoebel S, ed. An Era in Cardiovascular Medicine. New York : Elsevier; 1991 : 45-70.

15. Zoghbi WA, Enriquez-Sarano M, Foster E, et al. Recommendations for evaluation of the severity of native valvular regurgitation with two-dimensional and Doppler echocardiography. J Am Soc Echocardiogr 2003;16:777–802 (27).

Abbreviations

aPTT:	Activated partial thromboplastin time
AC:	Aortic closing sound
A2:	Aortic component of second heart sound
AF:	Atrial Fibrillation
AI:	Aortic insufficiency / Aortic incompetence
AO:	Aorta / Aortic opening sound
AR:	Aortic Regurgitation
AS:	Aortic Stenosis
AV:	Aortic Valve / Atrioventricular Valve
AVG:	Aortic valve gradient
AVA:	Aortic Valve Area
AVR:	Aortic valve replacement
BAV:	Balloon aortic valvotomy
BID:	Twice a Day (Lat: bis in die)
BMV:	Balloon mitral valvotomy
BPV:	Balloon pulmonary valvotomy
CC:	Closing click
CCL:	Counter clockwise loop
CABG:	Coronary artery bypass graft surgery
CAD:	Coronary artery disease
CCF:	Congestive cardiac failure
CE:	Cardiac enlargement
CHD:	Congenital heart disease
CHF:	Congestive heart failure
CNS:	Central Nervous System
DBP:	Diastolic Blood pressure
D/D:	Differential diagnosis
DVR:	Double Valve Replacement
DVI:	Doppler velocity index
EC:	Ejection click
ECG:	Electrocardiogram
EDM:	Early diastolic murmur
EF:	Ejection fraction
EMF:	Endomyocardial fibrosis
EOA:	Effective orifice area

E/O:	Evidence of
ERO:	Effective regurgitant orifice
ESD:	End systolic diameter
ESM:	Ejection systolic murmur
F/U:	Follow up
HCM:	Hypertrophic cardiomyopathy
HOCM:	Hypertrophic obstructive cardiomyopathy
IAS:	Interatrial septum
IE:	Infective endocarditis
IHJ	Indian Heart Journal
IM:	Intra-muscular
INR:	International normalized ratio
IRBBB:	Incomplete right bundle branch block
IU:	International units
IV:	Intra-venous
IVC:	Inferior vena cava
IVS:	Inter ventricular septum
JVP:	Jugular venous pulse
LA:	Left atrium
LAE:	Left atrial enlargement
LAD:	Left axis deviation
LAP:	Left atrial pressure
LBB:	Left bundle branch
LBBB:	Left bundle branch block
LCX:	Left circumflex
LDH:	Lactic Dehydrogenase
LICS:	Left intercostal space
LMWH:	Low molecular weight heparin
LSB:	Left sterna border
LV:	Left ventricle
LVEF:	Left ventricular ejection fraction
LVEDP:	Left ventricular end diastolic pressure
LVF:	Left ventricular failure
LVH:	Left ventricular hypertrophy
LVID:	LV internal Diameter

LVIDS:	LV internal Diameter in Systole
LVIDD:	LV internal Diameter in Diastole
LVSP:	Left ventricular systolic pressure
LVOT:	Left ventricle outflow tract
LVVO:	Left ventricular volume overload
M1:	Mitral component of S1
MC:	Mitral closing sound
MO:	Mitral opening sound
MR:	Mitral Regurgitation
MS:	Mitral stenosis
MV:	Mitral Valve
MDM:	Mid diastolic murmur
MVA:	Mitral valve area
MVP:	Mitral valve prolapse
MVR:	Mitral valve replacement
NYHA:	New York Heart Association
OC:	Opening click
OS:	Opening snap
OMV:	Open Mitral valvotomy
OTV:	Open tricuspid valvotomy
P2:	Pulmonary component of second heart sound
PA:	Pulmonary artery
PAH:	Pulmonary arterial hypertension
PAO2:	Pulmonary artery oxygen saturation
PASP:	Pulmonary artery systolic pressure
PAWP:	Pulmonary artery wedge pressure
PBMV:	Percutaneous Balloon Mitral Valvotomy
PDA:	Patent ductus arteriosus
PH:	Pulmonary hypertension
PHT:	Pressure half time
PND:	Paroxysmal nocturnal dyspnea
PO:	Per oral
PP:	Pulse pressure
PPM:	Prosthesis-Patient Mismatch
PS:	Pulmonary stenosis

PSA: Presystolic accentuation
PSM: Pansystolic murmur
PV: Pulmonary valve
PVE: Prosthetic valve endocarditis
PR: Pulmonary regurgitation
RA: Right atrium
RAE: Right atrial enlargement
RAP: Right atrial pressure
RBBB: Right bundle branch block
RBC: Red blood cell
RF: Regurgitant fraction
RHD: Rheumatic heart disease
RHF: Right heart failure
RV: Right ventricle
RV: Regurgitant volume
RVEF: Right ventricular ejection fraction
RVEDP: Right ventricular end diastolic pressure
RVH: Right ventricular hypertrophy
RVSP: Right ventricular systolic pressure
Rx: Treatment
S1:   First heart sound
S2:   Second heart sound
S3:   Third heart sound
S4:   Third heart sound
SBP: Systolic Blood pressure
SC: Subcutaneous
SCD: Sudden cardiac death
SLE: Systemic lupus erythematous
SM: Systolic murmur
T1:   Tricuspid component of S1
TEE: Trans esophageal echocardiography
TMT: Treadmill Test
TOF: Tetralogy Of Fallot
TTE: Trans thoracic echocardiography
TR: Tricuspid Regurgitation

TS:	Tricuspid stenosis
TMG:	Tricuspid mean gradient
TTG:	Tricuspid trans gradient
TV:	Tricuspid valve
UFH:	Unfractionated Heparin
VSD:	Ventricular septal defect
VTI:	Velocity time integral

About the Author

The author is an interventional cardiologist. He has completed his cardiology training from prestigious G S Seth Medical college and KEM Hospital, Mumbai, India. He has worked as cardiology fellow in Glasgow Royal Infirmary, Glasgow for 1 year. After completion of fellowship he has been practicing cardiology in Gujarat, India for last ten years. He has vast experience in Coronary as well as Rheumatic heart disease (RHD). RHD is still quite common in India and is a major cause of admission in hospitals. The author has rich experience of balloon valvuloplasties. His experience in dealing with valvular heart disease gives him an edge in writing a detailed book about multivalvular and prosthetic valve disease. In his series of handbooks about valve disease, he has already published "A Handbook of Rheumatic Fever", "A Handbook of Aortic valve disease and "A Handbook of Tricuspid and Pulmonary Valve disease". All these books have been published by Authorhouse. Apart from this handbook he has been a co-author of a book called "Patel's Atlas on Transradial Interventions: The basics" and has contributed as an author in "Patel's atlas on Transradial Interventions: Basics and Beyond". This handbook deals about the disease in great details. This handbook will be a very good reference book for students as well as medical practitioners.

www.ingramcontent.com/pod-product-compliance
Lightning Source LLC
Chambersburg PA
CBHW051419280526
45785CB00003B/1081